T0227251

Minimally Invasive Surgery in Orthopedic Surgery

Guest Editor

NICOLA MAFFULLI, MD, MS, PhD, FRCS (ORTH)

ORTHOPEDIC CLINICS OF NORTH AMERICA

www.orthopedic.theclinics.com

October 2009 • Volume 40 • Number 4

SAUNDERS an imprint of ELSEVIER, Inc.

W.B. SAUNDERS COMPANY
A Division of Elsevier Inc.

1600 John F. Kennedy Blvd. • Suite 1800 • Philadelphia, PA 19103-2899.

http://www.orthopedic.theclinics.com

ORTHOPEDIC CLINICS OF NORTH AMERICA Volume 40, Number 4
October 2009 ISSN 0030-5898, ISBN-10: 1-4377-1253-3, ISBN-13: 978-1-4377-1253-7

Editor: Deb Dellapena
Developmental Editor: Donald Mumford

Orthopedic Clinics of North America (ISSN 0030-5898) is published quarterly (For Post Office use only: Volume 40 issue 4 of 4) by Elsevier Inc., 360 Park Avenue South, New York, NY 10010-1710. Months of publication are January, April, July, and October. Subscription prices are $244.00 per year for (US individuals), $424.00 per year for (US institutions), $288.00 per year (Canadian individuals), $508.00 per year (Canadian institutions), $355.00 per year (international individuals), $508.00 per year (international institutions), $122.00 per year (US students), $177.00 per year (Canadian and international students). Foreign air speed delivery is included in all *Clinics* subscription prices. All prices are subject to change without notice. **POSTMASTER:** Send address changes to *Orthopedic Clinics of North America*, Elsevier Health Sciences Division, Subscription Customer Service, 3251 Riverport Lane, Maryland Heights, MO 63043. **Customer Service: 1-800-654-2452 (US and Canada). From outside of the United States and Canada, call 314-447-8871. Fax: 314-417-8029. E-mail: JournalsCustomerService-usa@elsevier.com (for print support); JournalsOnlineSupportusa@elsevier.com (for online support).**

Reprints. For copies of 100 or more, of articles in this publication, please contact the Commercial Reprints Department, Elsevier Inc., 360 Park Avenue South, New York, NY 10010-1710. Tel.: 212-633-3812; Fax: 212-462-1935; Email: reprints@elsevier.com.

Orthopedic Clinics of North America is covered in *MEDLINE/PubMed (Index Medicus), Cinahl, Excerpta Medica,* and *Cumulative Index to Nursing and Allied Health Literature.*

Printed and bound by CPI Group (UK) Ltd, Croydon, CR0 4YY

Transferred to Digital Print 2011

Contributors

GUEST EDITOR

NICOLA MAFFULLI,
MD, MS, PhD, FRCS (Orth)
Centre Lead and Professor of Sports and
Exercise Medicine, Consultant Trauma and
Orthopaedic Surgeon, Centre for Sports and
Exercise Medicine, Barts and The London
School of Medicine and Dentistry, Queen Mary
University of London, Mile End Hospital,
London, United Kingdom

AUTHORS

ERHAN BASAD, MD, PhD
Department of Orthopaedic Surgery, Giessen
University Hospital; Associate Medical
Director, Clinic & Polyclinic for Orthopaedic
Surgery, University Hospital Giessen-Marburg,
Germany

THOMAS BAUER, MD
Groupe de Recherche en Chirurgie
Mini-Invasive du Pied, Department of
Orthopaedic Surgery, Sport Medical Center,
Merignac; Department of Orthopaedic
Surgery, Ambroise Paré Hospital, West Paris
University, Boulogne, France

NICOLA BIASCA, MD
Head of Orthopaedic Surgery and Sport
Medicine Clinic, Co-Head of Trauma Surgery,
Department of Surgery, Spital Oberengadin,
Samedan (St. Moritz), Switzerland

DAVID BIAU, MD
Groupe de Recherche en Chirurgie
Mini-Invasive du Pied, Department of
Orthopedic Surgery, Sport Medical Center,
Merignac; Department of Orthopaedic
Surgery, Ambroise Paré Hospital, West Paris
University, Boulogne, France

LODOVICO RENZI BRIVIO, MD
Chief, Department of Orthopaedic and
Traumatology, C. Poma Hospital, Mantua, Italy

MATTHIAS BUNGARTZ, MD
Staff Member of Orthopaedic Surgery, Sports
Medicine and Trauma Surgery Clinic,
Department of Surgery, Spital Oberengadin,
Samedan (St. Moritz), Switzerland

ROBERTO CAUDANA, MD
Chief, Department of Radiology, C. Poma
Hospital, Mantua, Italy

PAOLO CELLOCCO, MD
Department of Orthopaedics, University
of Roma La Sapienza, Polo Pontino,
Istituto Chirurgico Ortopedico
Traumatologico, Italy

CRISTIANO COPPOLA, MD
Department of Orthopaedic Surgery, Ospedale
Loreto Mare, Napoli, Italy

GIUSEPPE COSTANZO, MD
Department of Orthopaedics, University of
Roma La Sapienza, Polo Pontino, Istituto
Chirurgico Ortopedico Traumatologico,
Italy

CHRISTOPHE DE LAVIGNE, MD
GRECMIP: Groupe de Recherche en Chirurgie Mini-Invasive du Pied, Department of Orthopaedic Surgery, Sport Medical Center, Merignac, France

LUCA DENARO, MD, PhD
Department of Neurosurgery, Catholic University School of Medicine, Policlinico Gemelli, Rome, Italy

VINCENZO DENARO, MD
Department of Orthopaedic and Trauma Surgery, Campus Biomedico University, Rome, Italy

MARIANO DE PRADO, MD
Groupe de Recherche en Chirurgie Mini-Invasive du Pied, Department of Orthopaedic Surgery, Sport Medical Center, Merignac, France; Hospital San Carlos, Murcia, Spain

GIAN LUCA DI TANNA, MSc, MPhil
Department of Experimental Medicine, University of Roma La Sapienza, Italy

STEFANO EL BOUSTANY, MD
Department of Orthopaedics, University of Roma La Sapienza, Polo Pontino, Istituto Chirurgico Ortopedico Traumatologico, Italy

NIKOLAOS GOUGOULIAS, MD, PhD, CCST(Ortho)
Clinical Fellow, Department of Trauma and Orthopaedic Surgery, Keele University School of Medicine, University Hospital of North Staffordshire, Staffordshire, United Kingdom

STEPHEN ISHAM, MD
Groupe de Recherche en Chirurgie Mini-Invasive du Pied, Department of Orthopaedic Surgery, Sport Medical Center, Merignac, France; Foot and Ankle Surgery Center, Coeur d'Alene, Idaho

BERND ISHAQUE, MD, PhD
Department of Orthopaedic Surgery, Giessen University Hospital; Assistant Medical Director, Clinic and Polyclinic for Orthopaedic Surgery, University Hospital Giessen-Marburg GmbH, Germany

JÖRG JEROSCH, MD, MD (Hon), PhD
Professor, Orthopaedic Department, Johanna-Etienne-Hospital Neuss; Medical Director, Clinic for Orthopaedics, Johanna-Etienne-Hospital, Neuss, Germany

ANIL KHANNA, MRCS, MS (Ortho)
Department of Trauma and Orthopaedic Surgery, Keele University School of Medicine, University Hospital of North Staffordshire; DePuy International Implant Research Fellow, University Hospital of North Staffordshire, Staffordshire, United Kingdom

OLIVIER LAFFENÊTRE, MD
Groupe de Recherche en Chirurgie Mini-Invasive du Pied, Department of Orthopaedic Surgery, Sport Medical Center, Merignac; Department of Orthopaedic Surgery, Bordeaux University Hospital, Bordeaux, France

UMILE GIUSEPPE LONGO, MD
Resident, Department of Orthopaedic and Trauma Surgery, Campus Biomedico University, Rome, Italy

NICOLA MAFFULLI, MD, MS, PhD, FRCS (Orth)
Centre Lead and Professor of Sports and Exercise Medicine, Consultant Trauma and Orthopaedic Surgeon, Centre for Sports and Exercise Medicine, Barts and The London School of Medicine and Dentistry, Queen Mary University of London, Mile End Hospital, London, United Kingdom

FRANCESCO OLIVA, MD, PhD
Staff Surgeon, Department of Orthopaedics and Traumatology, University of Rome Tor Vergata School of Medicine, Rome, Italy

NICOLA PAPAPIETRO, MD
Department of Orthopaedic and Trauma Surgery, Campus Biomedico University, Rome, Italy

ANDREA L. PIZZOLI, MD
Department of Orthopaedic and Traumatology, C. Poma Hospital, Mantua, Italy

MARIO RONGA, MD
Assistant Professor, Department of
Orthopaedic and Trauma Surgery, University
of Insubria, Varese, Italy

COSTANTINO ROSSI, MD
Division of Orthopaedics, Ospedali Riuniti
della Marsica, Tagliacozzo, Italy

THOMAS-OLIVER SCHNEIDER, MD
Head, Department of Orthopaedics,
Hirslanden Clinic Permanence, Bern; Former
Staff Member of Orthopaedic Clinic, Samedan
(St. Moritz), Switzerland

CHEZHIYAN SHANMUGAM, MD
Depuy International Fellow, Department of
Trauma and Orthopaedic Surgery, Keele
University School of Medicine, North

Staffordshire Hospital, Staffordshire, England,
United Kingdom

HENNING STÜRZ, MD, PhD
Professor, Department of Orthopaedic
Surgery, Giessen University Hospital; Medical
Director, Clinic and Polyclinic for Orthopaedic
Surgery, University Hospital Giessen-Marburg,
Germany

ENRICO VITTORINI, MD
Physician, Department of Radiology, C. Poma
Hospital, Mantua, Italy

TERRY L. WHIPPLE, MD
Chief of American Self Orthopaedics and
Director of Orthopaedic Research of Virginia,
Richmond, Virginia

Contents

tenuous blood supply and increased chance of wound breakdown and infection. This article presents recent advances in the field of minimally invasive AT surgery for tendinopathy, acute ruptures, and chronic tears. All of the techniques described in this article are inexpensive and do not require highly specialized equipment and training. Future randomized controlled trials are required to address the issue of the comparison between open versus minimally invasive AT surgery.

Minimally Invasive Osteosynthesis of Distal Tibial Fractures Using Locking Plates   499

Mario Ronga, Chezhiyan Shanmugam, Umile Giuseppe Longo, Francesco Oliva, and Nicola Maffulli

The management of distal tibia fractures can be challenging because of the scarcity of soft tissue, their subcutaneous nature, and poor vascularity. Classic open reduction and internal plate fixation require extensive soft tissue dissection and periosteal stripping, with high rates of complications. Minimally invasive plating techniques reduce iatrogenic soft tissue injury and damage to bone vascularity and preserve the osteogenic fracture hematoma. Locking plates (LPs) have the biomechanical properties of internal and external fixators, with superior holding power because of fixed angular stability through the head of locking screws, independent of friction fit. In this review, the rationale for the use of LPs and a description of the technique of minimally invasive LP osteosynthesis of distal tibia fractures are presented.

Percutaneous Hallux Valgus Surgery: A Prospective Multicenter Study of 189 Cases   505

Thomas Bauer, Christophe de Lavigne, David Biau, Mariano De Prado, Stephen Isham, and Olivier Laffenêtre

Distal first metatarsal osteotomies have been indicated for the correction of mild-to-moderate hallux valgus deformity. The aim of this study was to assess the clinical and radiographic results of the distal Reverdin–Isham first metatarsal osteotomy with use of a percutaneous procedure after a minimum 1-year followup. One hundred eighty-nine feet in 168 consecutive subjects were included in the present prospective multicenter study. A radiographic and clinical assessment using the American Orthopaedic Foot and Ankle Society's (AOFAS) hallux-metatarsophalangeal-interphalangeal scale was performed for all the subjects with a minimum 1-year follow-up. One hundred fifty six subjects (87%) were satisfied or very satisfied with the outcome of the procedure. The median postoperative AOFAS score was 93 points. Subjects averaged a loss 17% of first metatarsophalangeal joint motion. The median hallux valgus angle and Intermetatarsal angle improved from 28° and 13° preoperatively, to 14° and 10° postoperatively, respectively. Percutaneous correction of mild-to-moderate hallux valgus deformity with the Reverdin–Isham osteotomy of the first metatarsal enables us to achieve clinical and radiographic results comparable to other percutaneous or open distal metatarsal osteotomies after 1-year follow-up.

Bosch Osteotomy and Scarf Osteotomy for Hallux Valgus Correction   515

Nicola Maffulli, Umile Giuseppe Longo, Francesco Oliva, Vincenzo Denaro, and Cristiano Coppola

Minimally invasive distal metatarsal osteotomies are becoming broadly accepted for correction of hallux valgus. We compared the duration of surgery, the length of hospital stay, the American Orthopaedic Foot and Ankle Society (AOFAS) score, and the Foot and Ankle Outcome Score (FAOS) in 36 patients who underwent a minimal incision subcapital osteotomy of the first metatarsal with 36 matched patients who had hallux valgus corrected by a scarf technique. The minimum follow-up was

2.1 years (mean, 2.5 years; range, 2.1–3.2 years). Patients having the osteotomy had similar AOFAS and FAOS scores with less operating time and earlier discharge. Less operative time may benefit the patients, and earlier discharge has financial implications for the hospital.

Orthopedic Clinics of North America

FORTHCOMING ISSUES

January 2010

**Autologous Techniques to Fill Bone Defects
for Acute Fractures and Nonunions**
Hans C. Pape, MD, and
Timothy Weber, MD,
Guest Editors

April 2010

**Evidence-Based Medicine
in Orthopaedic Surgery**
Safdar N. Khan, MD, Mark A. Lee, MD,
and Munish C. Gupta, MD, *Guest Editors*

July 2010

Shoulder Instability
William N. Levine, MD, *Guest Editor*

October 2010

Orthopedic Management of Cerebral Palsy
Hank Chambers, MD, *Guest Editor*

RECENT ISSUES

July 2009

The Anterior Approach for Hip Reconstruction
Paul E. Beaulé, MD, FRCSC,
Guest Editor

April 2009

Bone Circulation Disorders
Michael A. Mont, MD, and
Lynne C. Jones, PhD,
Guest Editors

January 2009

Spine Oncology
Rakesh Donthineni, MD, MBA,
and Onder Ofluoglu, MD,
Guest Editors

THE CLINICS ARE NOW AVAILABLE ONLINE!

Access your subscription at:
www.theclinics.com

Preface

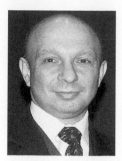

Nicola Maffulli, MD, MS, PhD, FRCS (Orth)
Guest Editor

Minimally invasive trauma and orthopedic surgery is increasingly taking hold. It is technically demanding. Although some would consider that arthroscopy is the ultimate minimally invasive procedure, over the course of the last few years many techniques and philosophies of treatment have been introduced and have since evolved. Now such techniques are used to manage fractures, nonunions, malunions, bone infections, arthritis, and deformities. These techniques have the theoretic advantage of decreasing recovery and rehabilitation times, because surgical exposure and deep tissue dissection are smaller and gentler to the soft tissues.

I have had the pleasure and privilege to work with seasoned innovators, and the result is a state-of-the-art collection of modern perspectives in this field. It is evident that to perform these techniques the surgeon has to be adept at the traditional ones. From a training viewpoint, it is still unclear what the learning curve is to be able to undertake these operations with a reliably high success rate. That many of the leaders in this field have matured through the traditional (and, some would say, maximally invasive) procedures to reach a position of preeminence in the minimally invasive movement speaks volumes.

This issue of *Orthopedic Clinics of North America* spans the whole body, from the upper to the lower limbs by way of the spine, hip, and knee. Not all the articles sing the praise of minimally invasive orthopedic surgery. The systematic review on minimally invasive total knee arthroplasty surgery

suggests that patients undergoing this procedure tend to experience decreased postoperative pain, rapid recovery of quadriceps function, reduced blood loss, improved range of motion (mostly reported as a short-term gain), and a shorter hospital stay compared with patients undergoing standard total knee arthroplasty. These benefits need to be balanced, however, against the incidence of increased tourniquet time and increased incidence of component malalignment in the minimally invasive total knee arthroplasty group. So far, the studies on minimally invasive orthopedic techniques are of moderate scientific quality with short follow-up periods. Multicenter studies with longer follow-up are needed to justify the long-term advantages of these techniques over traditional ones. Nevertheless, they are here to stay; let us have a glimpse at this brave new world.

Nicola Maffulli, MD, MS, PhD, FRCS (Orth)
Centre Lead and Professor of Sports
and Exercise Medicine
Consultant Trauma and Orthopaedic Surgeon
Centre for Sports and Exercise Medicine
Barts and The London School of Medicine and Dentistry
Mile End Hospital
275 Bancroft Road
London E1 4DG
England

E-mail address:
n.maffulli@qmul.ac.uk (N. Maffulli)

Orthop Clin N Am 40 (2009) xiii
doi:10.1016/j.ocl.2009.06.008
0030-5898/09/$ – see front matter © 2009 Elsevier Inc. All rights reserved.

orthopedic.theclinics.com

Dedication

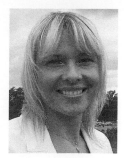
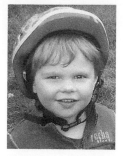

Gayle Denise Maffulli, BA(Hons)   Giuseppe D.P. Maffulli

I would like to dedicate this issue to Gayle Denise Maffulli, my wife, who has always been more than extremely supportive, and to Giuseppe Darius Peter Maffulli, my son, who inspires me each and every single day, though he does not sleep!

Nicola Maffulli, MD, MS, PhD, FRCS (Orth)
Centre Lead and Professor of Sports
and Exercise Medicine
Consultant Trauma and Orthopaedic Surgeon

Centre for Sports and Exercise Medicine
Barts and The London School
of Medicine and Dentistry
Mile End Hospital
275 Bancroft Road
London E1 4DG England

E-mail address:
n.maffulli@qmul.ac.uk (N. Maffulli)

Orthop Clin N Am 40 (2009) xv
doi:10.1016/j.ocl.2009.07.001

Dedication

Gayle Denise Maffulli, BA(Hons)   Giuseppe D.P. Maffulli

I would like to dedicate this issue to Gayle Denise Maffulli, my wife, who has always been more than extremely supportive, and to Giuseppe Darius Peter Maffulli, my son, who inspires me each and every single day, though he does not sleep!

Nicola Maffulli, MD, MS, PhD, FRCS (Orth)
Centre Lead and Professor of Sports
and Exercise Medicine
Consultant Trauma and Orthopaedic Surgeon

Centre for Sports and Exercise Medicine
Barts and The London School
of Medicine and Dentistry
Mile End Hospital
275 Bancroft Road
London E1 4DG England

E-mail address:
n.maffulli@qmul.ac.uk (N. Maffulli)

Orthop Clin N Am xx (2009) xx
doi:10.1016/j.ocl.2009.02.001
0030-5898/09/$ - see front matter © 2009 Elsevier Inc. All rights reserved.

orthopedic.theclinics.com

Minimally Invasive Carpal Tunnel Release

Paolo Cellocco, MD[a],*, Costantino Rossi, MD[b],
Stefano El Boustany, MD[a], Gian Luca Di Tanna, MSc, MPhil[c],
Giuseppe Costanzo, MD[a]

KEYWORDS

- Carpal tunnel release • Limited incision
- Mini-invasive surgery • KnifeLight
- Median nerve • Transverse carpal ligament

Carpal tunnel syndrome (CTS) is the most common compressive neuropathy in the upper extremity, with an incidence estimated at 3.46 per 1000.[1] It results from median nerve compression at the wrist, but increased intracarpal canal pressure may be a factor also. These conditions affect median nerve perfusion and produce the classic symptoms, including numbness, tingling, and weakness.[2] Occupational habits and gender are considered the most important risk factor for CTS, with a male-to-female ratio of 1 to 4.[3]

Open release of the transverse carpal ligament is classically performed through an extended longitudinal incision from the Kaplan cardinal line to the wrist crease or beyond.[4,5] This approach makes it possible to address additional conditions, such as displaced carpal fractures, osteophytes, and ganglions.[6]

Complications with the open technique include scar discomfort and tenderness, delayed healing, cosmetic complaints,[6–8] and weakening of pinch grip strength, which may be due to section of the interthenar fascia.[7] Palmar scar sensitivity is called pillar pain.

Several mini-invasive techniques have been introduced to avoid such complications and allow early recovery. With mini-invasive procedures, subcutaneous tissues are not widely dissected, potentially overcoming neuropathic pain complications.[9] Endoscopic procedures[10–13] decrease postoperative morbidity and accelerate patients' return to their activities of daily living. Endoscopic techniques require expensive equipment, however, with increased surgical time and a relatively long learning curve. Some complications may arise with this technique. For example, incomplete division of the transverse carpal ligament with increased rate of recurrence of CTS has been reported.[11–14] A cadaver study[15] showed incomplete release of the transverse carpal ligament with endoscopic procedures in 38% of specimens. Both mini-open and endoscopic techniques leave the interthenar fascia intact, which may be important in preserving pinch strength.[16]

Some investigators therefore prefer open approaches, by way of a short incision (palmar or carpal) and perform median nerve decompression either in a limited-open or mini-open, blind manner.[17–21] Limited-open techniques[5,18,21] are considered the standard procedure for carpal tunnel release (CTR).[22] Direct visualization of the whole transverse carpal ligament is achieved through a short (3–4 cm long) longitudinal incision. Section of the transverse carpal ligament is performed using generic tools, such as scalpels or scissors.

Avci and Sayli[17] described a minimally invasive technique using a short longitudinal palmar incision and a new knife, reporting good results with few complications. Skin incision, followed by the

[a] Department of Orthopedics, University of Roma "La Sapienza" – Polo Pontino, Istituto Chirurgico Ortopedico Traumatologico, via Franco Faggiana 1668, 04100 Latina, Italy
[b] Division of Orthopaedics, Ospedali Riuniti della Marsica, Presidio Ospedaliero di Tagliacozzo, via Variante, 67069 Tagliacozzo (AQ), Italy
[c] Department of Experimental Medicine, University of Roma "La Sapienza", viale Regina Elena 324, 00161 Roma, Italy
* Corresponding author.
E-mail address: paolo.cellocco@libero.it (P. Cellocco).

Orthop Clin N Am 40 (2009) 441–448
doi:10.1016/j.ocl.2009.06.002
0030-5898/09/$ – see front matter © 2009 Elsevier Inc. All rights reserved.

division of subcutaneous tissues, was made to visualize the distal edge of the flexor retinaculum; the knife was then directed in a distal-to-proximal direction to perform a blind retinaculum division.

Bhattacharaya and colleagues[23] performed a randomized controlled trial using the same knife used by Avci and Sayli[17] and open CTR to assess the potential advantages of this tool in terms of less scar tenderness and pillar pain; no significant differences were found. Another randomized study evaluating the same knife in 39 patients showed encouraging preliminary results.[24]

Our own technique involves a mini-open approach through a transverse incision less than 2 cm long at the distal crease of the wrist (**Fig. 1**). Through this incision, we directly visualize the proximal edge of the transverse carpal ligament, which we blindly divide with the KnifeLight used by Avci and Sayli. This instrument has its blade placed between two blunt plastic skids (KnifeLight, Stryker Instruments, Kalamazoo, Michigan). The KnifeLight has an integrated light source, which allows one to exactly locate the blade within deep tissues by transillumination.

The Boston Carpal Tunnel questionnaire (BCT), which is a patient-oriented, self-administered standardized instrument with good reproducibility and validity,[25,26] has been used to measure patient outcomes. The Italian modified version (BCTi) of this questionnaire has been validated.[26] It includes two sections, the first concerning symptoms evaluation (Symptoms Severity Scale). The first section is composed of 11 items, each item ranging from 1 (mild) to 5 (severe); the second section of the questionnaire investigates hand functions (Functional Status Scale), scoring 8 daily activities from 1 (no difficulty) to 5 (cannot perform the activity). The BCTi score modifications showed no correlation with nerve conduction values,

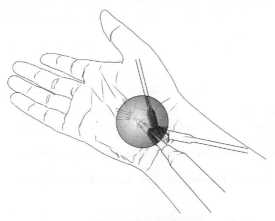

Fig. 1. Drawing shows the KnifeLight technique. (*Courtesy of* Elena Casagrande, Latina, Italy.)

measured both preoperatively and postoperatively.[27–29]

We report the long-term safety and effectiveness of the mini-incision CTR by way of blind transverse carpal ligament division with KnifeLight instrument compared with a standard open technique.

MATERIALS AND METHODS
Patients

From November 1999 to May 2001, 222 CTR procedures were performed on 185 consecutive patients. All patients gave their informed consent and were randomly divided into two groups by a simple coin toss (real or virtual on www.random.org). We randomized patients, not hands, as it would have complicated statistical analysis in some instances. Furthermore, this study did not address bilateral carpal tunnel syndrome as the study object, so we did not use patients who had bilateral procedures as their own control.

Neither patients nor the surgeon were blinded to the present study, because of the different incisions performed in this investigation. We compared patients in the two groups regarding gender, handedness, occupational status, distal motor latency, mean static two-point discrimination, and preoperative BCTi scores. There were no statistically significant differences in preoperative data between the two groups (**Table 1**). No patient received any workers' compensation.

Group A patients underwent the mini-open, blind technique using the KnifeLight instrument and Group B patients underwent the limited-open technique. The mean age was 59 years, ranging from 29 to 85 years. A total of 144 surgeries were performed on the right hand and 78 on the left hand. Group A included 82 patients and Group B included 103 patients. Ninety-nine procedures were performed in Group A, whereas 123 procedures were performed in Group B. There were 63 women and 19 men in Group A (mean age 60 years, range: 29–82), and 31 men and 72 women in Group B (mean age 59 years, range: 31–85). Differences in the size of the groups are due to the randomization process we used: coin toss does not split the study population in two equal parts, but is still a good and simple randomization tool.

Clinical evaluation and electrodiagnostic tests concurred for CTS diagnosis. Symptoms most frequently encountered were paraesthesia, which were found in 51 patients (62%) in Group A and in 58 patients (57%) in Group B; hypoesthesia, which was found in 36 patients (43%) in Group A and in 50 patients (49%) in Group B; and nocturnal

Table 1
Results of the Italian modified version of the Boston Carpal Tunnel questionnaire

		Group A n = 99	Group B n = 123	ANOVA	t test
1st section	Preoperative	3.85 (0.75)	3.67 (0.71)	—	0.0651
	19 mo	1.46 (0.52)	2.05 (0.82)	—	<0.001
	30 mo	1.28 (0.59)	1.39 (0.72)	0.0424	0.233
	60 mo	1.33 (0.64)	1.38 (0.83)	0.0424	0.629
2nd section	Preoperative	3.87 (0.75)	3.80 (0.77)	—	0.4843
	19 mo	2.02 (0.82)	2.54 (0.88)	—	<0.001
	30 mo	1.88 (0.75)	1.73 (0.83)	0.4835	0.1715
	60 mo	1.80 (0.78)	1.75 (0.97)	0.4835	0.678

Table shows mean BCTi scores in Group A and B, ANOVA, and Student t test P values preoperatively and at 19, 30, and 60 months' follow-up. SD is shown in parentheses.

Modified from Cellocco P, Rossi C, Bizzarri F, et al. mini-open blind procedure versus limited-open technique for carpal tunnel release: a 30-months follow-up study. J Hand Surg 2005;30-A:493–99; with permission.

waking, which was found in 31 patients (38%) in Group A and in 53 patients (52%) in Group B. Preoperative mean static two-point discrimination score was evaluated using a caliper (a handmade modified common hardware tool); the mean score was 7.2 mm in Group A patients (SD = 0.925; range: 6–9 mm) and 7.6 mm for patients in Group B (SD = 1.069; range: 6–10 mm). The minimum duration of symptoms was 6.3 months (range: 2–15 months) for patients in Group A, whereas patients in Group B had experienced symptoms for a mean duration of 7.7 months (range: 3–14 months). The index and long fingers were the most affected (164 of 222 hands, 74%), and 80 of 222 (36%) patients complained of pain at the forearm or elbow. Eighty-one hands in Group A (82%) and 97 hands in Group B (79%) had a positive Phalen test. A positive Tinel sign was found in 91 hands in Group A (92%) versus 118 hands in Group B (96%). Noticeable thenar hypotrophy was found in 8 hands in Group A (8%) and 14 hands (11%) in Group B. Following the classification proposed by Padua and colleagues[20,27] all patients were considered to have mild to moderate median nerve compression at the wrist. Median nerve distal motor latency ranged from 4.5 to 6.8 milliseconds for patients in Group A (mean = 5.9 milliseconds, SD = 0.6) and from 4.7 to 7.1 milliseconds for patients in Group B (mean = 6.0 milliseconds, SD = 0.6).

The Italian modified version of the Boston Carpal Tunnel (BCTi) questionnaire[25,26] was self-administered preoperatively to all patients, and then readministered after a mean follow-up of 19 months (range: 12–28 months), 30 months (range: 24–42 months), and at the last outpatient appointment (minimum follow-up: 60 months, range: 60 to 87 months). Patients answered both sections of the questionnaire, which respectively evaluate

hand symptoms and hand function. No electrodiagnostic test was performed at the follow-up, except when recurrent median nerve was suspected. Mean static two-point discrimination score was re-evaluated with the same follow-up scheduling as BCTi scores. At the 30-months and 60-months office appointments, patients were asked to subjectively grade their cosmetic results from poor to excellent (poor: totally unsatisfied; fair: partially satisfied; good: only slightly unsatisfied; excellent: totally satisfied). We evaluated complications and symptoms recurrence rates.

Surgical Technique

The senior author (GC) performed study procedures in an outpatient setting, with an axillary block or local anesthesia. We recorded operating times for each procedure in the two groups. In Group A, we used the tourniquet in all but two patients (those who had local anesthesia). A towel roll was used to place the wrist in moderate extension. A short transverse incision, 1.5 to 2 cm long, was performed at the distal crease of the wrist (**Fig. 2**). The antebrachial fascia was divided, and the proximal edge of the transverse carpal ligament and insertions of the palmaris longus tendon were directly visualized. Using a scalpel, a 5-mm longitudinal incision was made on the proximal edge of the retinaculum until the median nerve became evident under the fibrous tissue. Care was taken not to damage the median nerve. The distal edge of the KnifeLight was then placed in this incision, under direct vision, with its long skid laying on the ulnar margin of the median nerve and the short skid overriding the carpal ligament. This placement insured the surgeon against the chance of incomplete division of the carpal

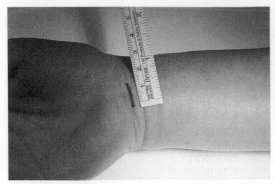

Fig. 2. The transverse incision at the distal crease of the wrist performed on Group A patients.

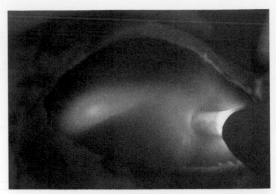

Fig. 4. When the spotlight becomes clearly visible under the skin, the transverse carpal ligament is divided.

ligament. The tool light was switched on, and the operative light switched off. At this time, a diffuse, pale light was seen through the skin of the palm (Fig. 3), probably due to the collagen fibers in the transverse carpal ligament absorbing light. The tool was then gently pushed forward, blindly directing it toward the third intermetacarpal space and keeping the blade toward the palmar surface of the hand, until the tissue resistance suddenly decreased and a bright, sharp-edged spotlight became clearly visible in the palmar region (Fig. 4), indicating complete ligament division. This phenomenon was due to lack of light absorption by collagen fibers because the transverse carpal ligament had been fully sectioned. A probe was then inserted into the carpal tunnel passing it through the skin incision to make sure that the carpal tunnel was completely opened. In eight subjects we performed a proximal release of the antebrachial fascia, because of strong adhesions of the fascia about the median nerve. In patients who had axillary block, the tourniquet was deflated and we inspected the wound, waiting 1 to 2

minutes, assessing integrity of the superficial palmar arch. In patients who had local anesthesia, the nerve function was assessed also, asking them to move the thumb. The skin incision was then closed with 3/0 or 4/0 monofilament nonabsorbable sutures.

A limited-open approach[5,18,21] was used in Group B patients (Fig. 5). In 122 of 123 procedures a tourniquet was used.[5] We started the incision at the Kaplan cardinal line, according to Steinberg's technique. The 3- to 4-cm long incision was made 3 to 4 mm ulnarly from the midline and parallel with the thenar crease, and was directed toward the ulnar border of the palmaris longus. We bluntly dissected the subcutaneous tissues and located the whole transverse carpal ligament.

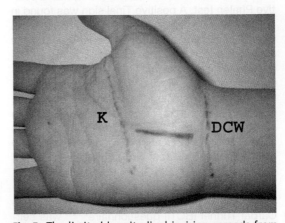

Fig. 5. The limited longitudinal incision spreads from the distal crease of the wrist (DCW) proximally to the Kaplan cardinal line distally (K). Note that the incision is directed toward the third intermetacarpal space. (From Cellocco P, Rossi C, Bizzarri F, et al. Mini-open blind procedure versus limited-open technique for carpal tunnel release: a 30-months follow-up study. J Hand Surg 2005;30-A:493–99; with permission.)

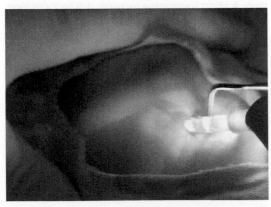

Fig. 3. With the light switched on, the instrument is gently directed in a proximal-distal direction.

The proximal edge of the transverse carpal ligament was carefully incised, and a blunt probe was inserted to protect the underlying median nerve. The transverse carpal ligament was then divided under direct vision using a scalpel or scissors. The tourniquet was deflated, and we performed a meticulous hemostasis. The subcutaneous tissues were not sutured. The skin incision was closed with 3/0 or 4/0 monofilament nonabsorbable sutures.

No postoperative splints were used, and patients were encouraged to use their hands normally. Heavy activities were avoided during the first three postoperative weeks. All patients were interviewed by telephone 30 days after surgery to assess their time to return to work.

Statistics

Data were entered in a commercially available database (Stata 10.2, StataCorp LP, College Station, Texas). Descriptive statistics were calculated. We compared preoperative and 19-month postoperative mean BCTi scores of each section in the questionnaire using Student t test and then compared preoperative and postoperative (30 and 60 months) scores by means of ANOVA for repeated measures. Significance was set at $P \leq 0.05$, with 95% confidence interval.

RESULTS

The mean operating time from skin incision to skin closure in Group A was always shorter than 20 minutes (mean = 16.24, SD = 4.15). The three anxious female patients with an operating time of about 35 minutes were clearly outliers. For Group B procedures, surgery duration was always more than 30 minutes (mean = 35.16, SD = 2.90). No early complications, vascular or neurologic, were observed in any patients. No patients dropped out of the study after 60 months' follow-up. In the postoperative evaluation, the two sections of BCTi were analyzed separately. The Student t test of postoperative values at mean follow-up of 19 months in each section of the BCTi questionnaire showed that patients in Group A had significantly better results than patients in Group B. ANOVA for repeated measures was used to assess differences between and within groups. At a mean follow-up of 30 months, these differences showed no significance. No significant differences were detected after a minimum follow-up of 60 months (see **Table 1**).

Patients in Group A returned to work in 16.6 days (range: 15–18 days), whereas patients in Group B returned to work in 25.4 days (range: 23–29 days) ($P < 0.001$).

At the 60-month follow-up the mean static two-point discrimination score was 4.6 mm for patients in Group A and 4.5 mm for patients in Group B. These differences were not statistically significant.

At the latest office appointment, eight hands (6.5%) in group B had clinical evidence of recurrent CTS, compared with three patients (3%) in Group A.

After a mean 30 months' follow-up, all patients in Group A were satisfied with their cosmetic results (100% good to excellent results). Subjective satisfaction with their scar was present in 96 hands of 82 patients (78% good to excellent results) in Group B. Nineteen patients (23 hands, 18.7%), in Group B had fair results, whereas 2 patients (4 hands, 3.3%) reported poor results. Ratings in Group B showed slight changes at the latest office appointment (60 months, mean), with 98 hands of 84 patients cosmetically considered as good to excellent, 20 hands (16 patients) considered fair, and 5 hands (3 patients) considered poor. At the latest follow-up appointment, all patients in Group A scored their cosmetic condition as good or excellent. In Group B 81 patients (95 hands), 21 patients (26 hands), and 1 patient (2 hands) had good to excellent, fair, and poor cosmetic results, respectively.

DISCUSSION

Surgery for CTR has evolved to decrease its already minimal complication rate. The classic procedure for the management of CTS is the open release of the transverse carpal ligament. The incision is long, and, in some instances, it heals with a tender scar. Some investigators use postoperative splinting.[6-8] Several attempts to lessen exposure size with limited-incision approaches have been proposed.[5,17-21,30]

Hand surgeons generally perform longitudinal incisions more than 4 cm in length in 65.8% of patients, whereas 31.9% of them prefer a longitudinal incision less than 4 cm and only 0.6% used a transverse incision.[4] Nathan and colleagues[20] compared CTRs performed using an incision greater than 2.5 cm and those performed with smaller incisions and concluded that "…the smaller the incision, the shorter was the recovery period."

Complaints related to incision length may be addressed by endoscopic procedures, which are well accepted by patients. Some anatomic considerations account for the theoretic advantages of endoscopic surgery. Da Silva[9] showed that it avoids disruption of unmyelinated nerve fibers at the interthenar crease originating from the palmar cutaneous branch of the median nerve, which lie in the superficial, loose connective tissue palmar to the flexor retinaculum. By contrast, there are no nerve fibers in the deep, dense collagen aspect of the ligament.

Leaving these branches intact makes it possible to avoid the development of microscopic neuromas and subsequent pain after standard CTR. Nevertheless, endoscopic CTR may lead to complications.[11–14] Anatomic abnormalities may be misdiagnosed intraoperatively, as we previously reported on a female patient who had CTS and a bifid median nerve, not previously recognized with endoscopic technique, who had CTS symptom recurrence.[31]

Most previous studies concerning different minimal invasive techniques report only short- or medium-term follow-up. The present investigation addresses this limit and extends our previous experience on a minimally invasive technique[32] from 30 to 60 months.

Blind mini-open procedures are being performed using a small longitudinal palmar incision[17] or a transverse wrist incision,[9,30–33] with no or few complications. Minimally invasive techniques allow earlier recovery of the function of the operated hand, even though medium- and long-term results show no significant differences between open, mini-incision, and endoscopic procedures.[19,23,24,32]

In a recent retrospective work, Lee and colleagues[34] reported on 1332 Indiana Tome (Biomet, Warsaw, IN) CTRs performed between 1993 and 2006, with an overall complication rate of 0.83%, confirming safety and effectiveness of blind instruments.

Another long-term study on Indiana Tome reported one intraoperative partial median nerve laceration and 9 of 100 patients the Indiana Tome group requiring further treatment. The recurrence rate was not statistically different when compared with the control group. It remains unclear whether the nerve damage should be attributed to the investigators' limited experience in this technique, and may account for the initial learning curve.[35]

The Safeguard System (Kyneticos Medical, San Diego, California) is a similar tool with two components, a blunt guide and a knife, used for CTR. No follow-up studies are available at the moment to our knowledge.[36]

There are several surgical tools to perform blind CTR, but the KnifeLight seems to be extremely safe,[17,32] with its blunt skids protecting the median nerve and the motor branch of the median nerve. The cutaneous branch (palmar cutaneous nerve), which lies on the radial side of the CT, is also protected. The integrated light source allows for better localization of the blade during division of the flexor retinaculum, avoiding vascular damage.[32]

Hwang and Ho[37] reported on 44 consecutive patients operated on with the KnifeLight, with excellent functional outcomes at a mean follow-up of 6 months.

The KnifeLight instrument does not allow direct visualization of the carpal tunnel content, which may be considered a disadvantage. Nevertheless, incomplete carpal tunnel decompression can be avoided by dividing the transverse carpal ligament fully, under direct visualization of the proximal edge of the carpal ligament.

Avci and Sayli[17] studied 31 wrists of 25 patients operated on with KnifeLight. To avoid the risk for inadvertently cutting the superficial palmar arch or incompletely releasing the transverse carpal ligament, they preferred an incision in the palmar region with ligament division directed proximally instead of a wrist incision with ligament division directed distally. Abouzahr and colleagues[30] performed release procedures on 28 cadavers with one palmar arch injured. Carter[33] used a CTR device similar to KnifeLight on 100 patients with no complications. A complete median nerve transection has been reported as a complication of CT release with a slightly different device.[38] This single case report described a female patient previously operated in an institution other than the author's. It is difficult to state whether this represents a high or a low complication rate for surgeons who first operated that patient.

Our experience in CT releases using a short wrist incision was based on blindly dividing the transverse carpal ligament simply with scissors or a scalpel. In our work, we now use the KnifeLight through the same transverse incision. We alternatively use limited longitudinal incisions,[5,18,19] which we performed on Group B patients in this study.

Potential damages during such a minimally invasive surgery may occur, and they include section of the superficial palmar arch. The superficial palmar arch is embedded in a fat pad, which preserves it from injuries. A safe blind procedure is performed when the knife is moderately angled toward the hand surface and directed toward the third intermetacarpal space. The division of the transverse carpal ligament is then stopped when ligament resistance suddenly decreases and a spotlight becomes clearly visible under the skin, indicating complete ligament division (see **Fig. 4**). Nevertheless, no branches arise from the median nerve at its ulnar side beneath or beyond the transverse carpal ligament, so that neural damage may be considered uneven.[39]

Postoperative wrist pain is believed to be more likely if the subcutaneous tissue at the wrist was dissected.[21] In our experience, inflammation and hematomas are lessened by limiting the incision length and leaving the subcutaneous volar space of the carpus undisturbed (remaining under the palmar fascia), thus avoiding postoperative tenderness in this area. A small but significant number of recurrences occurred in the present study among Group B patients (seven patients, 5%), whereas only one patient (<1%) in Group A had clinical signs of recurrence ($P < 0.01$). These data have been confirmed in a study by Klein and colleagues.[40]

Incisions at the proximal crease of the wrist may not provide the opportunity to directly visualize the neurovascular structures located in the palmar region, thus increasing the risk for damaging them. Nevertheless, a careful proximal approach is safe, especially when the transverse carpal ligament is gently divided with the tool used in this study. The learning curve for this surgical technique is relatively short, especially for surgeons who are used to performing CTRs with open techniques. Eventually, further studies are needed to definitively assess anatomic consequences of this technique.

Vascular and neurologic complications can be avoided with knowledge of the anatomy of the CT, thus preserving the structures at risk. A safe method to use the blind technique that we previously proposed[32] is to gently push the knife toward the third intermetacarpal space and to stop after division of the transverse carpal ligament.

In patients undergoing minimally invasive procedures, normal activities were generally resumed shortly after surgery, and return to work was possible in 15 to 18 days (mean: 16.6 days). By contrast, patients treated with limited-open surgery resume their previous occupational activities after 23 to 29 days (mean: 25.4 days). These data are highly significant ($P < 0.001$), and should be considered when dealing with patients in need of a faster recovery.

Our experience suggests that minimally invasive CT release may be safely performed using a small transverse wrist incision. The BCTi questionnaire showed better outcomes in patients treated with the blind technique than those treated with limited-open procedures in the short term. The differences between the two groups tend to be less evident at medium- and long-term follow-up, and after a mean follow-up of 30 and 60 months from surgery, the two procedures are equally effective in relieving symptoms in patients who have carpal tunnel syndrome. Finally, patients were subjectively more satisfied from a cosmetic viewpoint with the minimally invasive technique.

ACKNOWLEDGEMENTS

The authors thank Prof. Annarita Vestri for helping with statistics and Miss Elena Casagrande for drawings.

REFERENCES

1. Nordstrom DL, Vierkant RA, DeStefano F, et al. Risk factors for carpal tunnel syndrome in a general population. Occup Environ Med 1997;54:734–40.

2. Franzblau A, Werner R. What is carpal tunnel syndrome? JAMA 1999;282:186–7.

3. Higgs PE, Edwards S, Martin DS, et al. Carpal tunnel surgery outcomes in workers: effect of worker's compensation status. J Hand Surg Am 1995;20: 354–60.

4. Duncan KH, Lewis RC, Foreman KA, et al. Treatment of carpal tunnel syndrome by members of the American Society for Surgery of the Hand: results of a questionnaire. J Hand Surg Am 1987;12:384–91.

5. Steinberg DR. Surgical release of the carpal tunnel. Hand Clin 2002;18:291–8.

6. Kessler FB. Complications of the management of carpal tunnel syndrome. Hand Clin 1986;2:401–6.

7. MacDonald RI, Lichtman DM, Hanlon JJ, et al. Complications of surgical release for carpal tunnel syndrome. J Hand Surg Am 1978;3:70–6.

8. Louis DS, Greene TL, Noellert R. Complications of carpal tunnel surgery. J Neurosurg 1985;65:352–6.

9. Da Silva MF, Moore DC, Weiss AP, et al. Anatomy of the palmar cutaneous branch of the median nerve: clinical significance. J Hand Surg Am 1996;21: 639–43.

10. Okutsu I, Ninomiya S, Takatori Y, et al. Endoscopic management of carpal tunnel syndrome. Arthroscopy 1989;5:11–8.

11. Chow JC. Endoscopic release of the carpal ligament for carpal tunnel syndrome: 22-month clinical result. Arthroscopy 1990;6:288–96.

12. Agee JM, McCarroll HR, Tortosa RD, et al. Endoscopic release of the carpal tunnel: a randomized prospective multicenter study. J Hand Surg Am 1992;17:987–95.

13. Brown RA, Gelberman RH, Seiler JH, et al. Carpal tunnel release. A prospective randomized assessment of open and endoscopic methods. J Bone Joint Surg Am 1993;75:1265–75.

14. Palmer AK, Toivonen DA. Complications of endoscopic and open carpal tunnel release. J Hand Surg Am 1999;24:561–5.

15. Rowland ED, Kleinert JM. Endoscopic carpal tunnel release in cadavera. J Bone Joint Surg Am 1994;76: 266–8.

16. Cobb TK, Cooney WP. Significance of incomplete release of the distal portion of the flexor retinaculum:

implications for endoscopic carpal tunnel surgery. J Hand Surg Am 1994;19:283–5.

17. Avci S, Sayli U. Carpal tunnel release using a short palmar incision and a new knife. J Hand Surg Br 2000;25:357–60.

18. Bromley GS. Minimal-incision open carpal tunnel decompression. J Hand Surg Am 1994;19:119–20.

19. Lee WP, Strickland JW. Safe carpal tunnel release via a limited palmar incision. Plast Reconstr Surg 1998;101(2):418–24.

20. Nathan PA, Meadows KD, Keniston RC. Rehabilitation of carpal tunnel surgery patients using a short surgical incision and an early program of physical therapy. J Hand Surg Am 1993;18:1044–50.

21. Serra JM, Benito JR, Monner J. Carpal tunnel release with short incision. Plast Reconstr Surg 1997;99(1):129–35.

22. Zyluk A, Strychar J. A comparison of two limited open techniques for carpal tunnel release. J Hand Surg Br 2006;31:466–72.

23. Bhattacharaya R, Birdsall PD, Stothard J. A randomized controlled trial of Knifelight and open carpal tunnel release. J Hand Surg Br 2004;29:113–5.

24. Helm RH, Vaziri S. Evaluation of carpal tunnel release using the Knifelight instrument. J Hand Surg Br 2003;28:251–4.

25. Levine D, Simmons B, Koris MJ, et al. A self-administered questionnaire for the assessment of severity of symptoms and functional status in carpal tunnel syndrome. J Bone Joint Surg Am 1993;75:1585–92.

26. Padua R, Padua L, Romanini E, et al. Versione italiana del questionario "Boston Carpal Tunnel": valutazione preliminare [Italian version of Boston Carpal Tunnel Questionnaire. Early evaluation]. Giornale Italiano di Ortopedia e Traumatologia 1998;24:121–9 [in Italian].

27. Mondelli M, Reale F, Sicurelli F, et al. Relationship between the self-administered Boston Questionnaire and electrophysiological findings in follow-up of surgically-treated carpal tunnel syndrome. J Hand Surg Br 2000;25:128–34.

28. Padua L, LoMonaco M, Gregori B, et al. Neurophysiological classification and sensitivity in 500 carpal

tunnel syndrome hands. Acta Neurol Scand 1997; 96:211–7.

29. Padua L, Padua R, Lo Monaco M, et al. Multiperspective assessment of carpal tunnel syndrome. Neurology 1999;53:1654–9.

30. Abouzahr MK, Patsis MC, Chiu DT. Carpal tunnel release using limited direct vision. Plast Reconstr Surg 1995;95(3):534–8.

31. Rossi C, Cellocco P, Costanzo G. Bifid median nerve as a determinant of carpal tunnel sindrome recurrence after endoscopic procedures. A case report. J Orthop Trauma 2003;4:92–4.

32. Cellocco P, Rossi C, Bizzarri F, et al. Mini-open blind procedure versus limited-open technique for carpal tunnel release: a 30-months follow-up study. J Hand Surg Am 2005;30:493–9.

33. Carter SL. A new instrument: a carpal tunnel knife. J Hand Surg Am 1991;16:178–9.

34. Lee WPA, Schipper BM, Goitz RJ. 13-year experience of carpal tunnel release using the Indiana Tome technique. J Hand Surg Am 2008;33: 1052–6.

35. Cresswell TR, Heras-Palou C, Bradley MJ, et al. Long-term outcome after carpal tunnel decompression – a prospective randomized study of the Indiana Tome and an standard limited palmar incision. J Hand Surg Eur Vol 2008;33:332–6.

36. Hughes TB, Baratz M. Limited open carpal tunnel syndrome using the Safeguard system. Tech Orthop 2006;21:12–8.

37. Hwang PYK, Ho CL. Minimally invasive carpal tunnel decompression using the KnifeLight. Neurosurgery 2007;60(2 Suppl 1):ONS162–8.

38. Chapman CB, Ristic S, Rosenwasser MP. Complete median nerve transection as a complication of carpal tunnel release with a carpal tunnel tome. Am J Orthop 2001;30:652–3.

39. Lanz U. Anatomical variation of the median nerve in the carpal tunnel. J Hand Surg Am 1977;2:44–53.

40. Klein RD, Kotsis SV, Chung KC. Open carpal tunnel release using a 1-centimeter incision: technique and outcomes for 104 patients. Plast Reconstr Surg 2003;11(5):1616–22.

Percutaneous CT-Guided Vertebroplasty in the Management of Osteoporotic Fractures and Dorsolumbar Metastases

Andrea L. Pizzoli, MD[a],*, Lodovico Renzi Brivio, MD[a],
Roberto Caudana, MD[b], Enrico Vittorini, MD[b]

KEYWORDS
- Spine vertebroplasty • Spine fractures • Spine CT
- Spine secondary neoplasms • Osteoporosis

Percutaneous vertebroplasty (PVP) is a minimally invasive, image-guided procedure consisting of an injection of acrylic cement into a vertebral body to reinforce the compressed segment and achieve pain relief. The first PVP was performed in Europe in 1984[1] and nearly a decade later (1993) in North America.[2] Initially used to treat aggressive vertebral hemangioma, PVP was later extended to other painful vertebral lesions caused by metastases, osteoporotic vertebral compression fractures, myeloma, and other less common conditions (histocytosis, osteogenesis imperfecta).[3] Since the earliest experiences, PVP has undergone numerous modifications; this has led to better results, shorter procedure times, and fewer complications.

We present our personal experience to describe the technique applied and report the results achieved in more than 100 patients who had PVP performed under CT guidance.[4]

MATERIALS AND METHODS

Our first published series consisted of 182 PVPs performed in 106 patients, 67 of whom had osteoporosis and 39 of whom had metastases. Patients who had osteoporosis underwent 120 PVP procedures, 93 of which were at the lumbar level (77.5%); patients who had metastasis underwent 62 PVPs, 35 of which were at the dorsal level (56.4%).[4]

Preoperative Assessment

Patient selection has been done by a multidisciplinary team (an internist specializing in metabolic bone disease, an oncologist, an orthopaedic surgeon, and a radiologist) following the guidelines suggested by American College of Radiology Standards 2000–2001.[5] Indications for PVP were dorsolumbar vertebral fractures due to recent osteoporotic vertebral collapse associated with pain resistant to medical therapy (rest, analgesics, orthopaedic corset) and dorsolumbar vertebral metastases with fractures or areas of vertebral body osteolysis without adequate response to medical therapy. Contraindications to PVP were involvement of the spinal canal by retropulsed fracture fragments or by tumor extension into the epidural space, severe vertebral collapse to less than one third of the original vertebral height, spondylodiscitis, hemorrhagic diathesis, and known allergies to any of the products used for the procedure (local anesthetic and acrylic cement).

[a] Orthopaedic and Traumatology Department, C. Poma Hospital, V. le Albertoni n1; 46100 Mantova, Italy
[b] Radiology Department, C. Poma Hospital, V. le Albertoni n1; 46100 Mantova, Italy
* Corresponding author.
E-mail address: andreapizzoli@hotmail.com (A.L. Pizzoli).

All patients were administered a 10-point visual analogue scale (10, worst ever pain; 1, no pain) for pain assessment,[6] a 4-point functional mobility scale (4, bedridden; 3, use of wheelchair; 2, limited painful ambulation; 1, normal ambulation) and a 3-point analgesic use scale (3, complete daily coverage; 2, partial daily coverage; 1, occasional coverage). Data from the above assessments were collected in a questionnaire.

All patients also underwent laboratory testing and radiographic assessment (anteroposterior and lateral radiograms and MRI). Radiographic and MRI examinations helped to determine patients' anatomic compatibility for PVP based on the following findings:

Evidence, on the lateral radiogram or midsagittal MR images, of vertebral collapse with at least one third of original height preserved, as shown by comparison with previous normal radiographs or MR images or, if unavailable, by measuring normal-appearing vertebral bodies adjacent to the collapsed one (**Fig. 1**)[7,8]

Evidence on the lateral radiogram or MR images of areas of osteolysis or vertebral body fracture with intact posterior wall, vertebral pedicles, and spinal canal

No MR evidence of spinal cord or nerve root compression

Signs of recent vertebral collapse with MR signal change due to bone marrow edema and characterized by T1 hypointensity and T2 hyperintensity enhanced by fat suppression (see **Fig. 1**)

Concordance between vertebral levels of the change in bone marrow signal and pain sites

Absence of contrast enhancement of the epidural tissue that indicates on MR images neoplastic spread of metastases

Absence of radiographic evidence of osteosclerosis of the vertebral trabecular network (secondary to spontaneous repair or induced by chemotherapy or radiotherapy) likely to hinder the introduction of cement into the vertebral body.

Instrumentation

In the major part of the procedures we used a Simko kit (Optimed, Ettlingen, Germany) composed of needles with stylet and bevel or diamond tip, 15-, 13-, and 10-gauge caliber and 10 to 15 cm long, a syringe with a manual injector, and attachments for the aspiration/injection of acrylic cement (**Fig. 2**). In all cases, we used the radiopaque acrylic cement Mendec Spine (Tecres

S.p.A., Sommacampagna, Verona, Italy) mainly composed of polymethylmethacrylate (PMMA) and with a polymerization time less than 10 minutes. The cement was prepared mixing the solvent (9.4 g of MMA, N,N-dimethyl-p-toluidine, hydroquinone) with the powder (20 g of PMMA, 30% barium sulphate, benzoyl peroxide) for 30 seconds in a closed bottle to avoid the formation of potentially toxic vapors.[9] With a 10-mL syringe we induced the local anesthesia using the needles included in the kit or Chiba needles (18–19 gauge, length 20 cm). These needles have been useful for deep anesthesia and as a guide to advance the PVP needle coaxially from the skin to the bone cortex, after cutting the external tip of the needle when necessary (plastic connector in the Chiba needles). Finally, we used a scalpel for the skin incision at the entry point and a 3-hg weight surgical hammer to help the needle penetrate the bone (**Fig. 3**).

Methods

Patients were informed about the benefits and risks of the procedure before providing their informed consent. To minimize the risk for infection, in agreement with the literature,[4,10] patients who were immunocompromised because of cancer therapy received antibiotic prophylaxis 3 days before the procedure. PVP was carried out under CT guidance in all cases. In our first series for the first 78 patients (135 PVP) we used a single-slice spiral CT (Picker PQ5000, Cleveland, Ohio) combined with conventional radiofluoroscopy (Siremobil Iso-C; Siemens, Erlangen, Germany); subsequently (28 patients for 47 PVP in the first series) we performed the procedure using a multislice spiral CT alone (Sensation 16; Siemens) with the following CT-fluoroscopy equipment:

An additional 17-in liquid-crystal monitor, placed inside the CT room and moveable to be well visualized by the operator, with identical capabilities to the monitor of the main console (**Fig. 4**A). This monitor allows real-time display of axial CT-fluoroscopy images and visualization of axial images acquired on the volume or reconstructed with multiplanar reformatting (MPR) in the sagittal and coronal planes. The operator could thus follow the most delicate phases of the procedure (needle placement in the vertebral body, cement injection) on the axial CT-fluoroscopy images in real time to evaluate cement distribution in the vertebra and identify immediately even the slightest cement leak, which requires

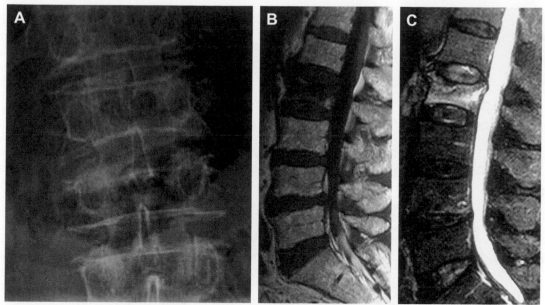

Fig. 1. A 64-year-old woman who had osteoporosis. Anatomic compatibility for PVP of L2. (*A*) In the anteroposterior radiographic view, compression fracture of the L2 vertebral body with height not less than one third of the original. Normal height of the other lumbar vertebral bodies. (*B, C*) Sagittal MR images obtained with turbo spin-echo T1-weighted (*B*) and fat-suppressed short tau inversion recovery (STIR) T2-weighted (*C*). Sequences show a change in signal intensity at the L2 vertebral body, characterized by T1 hypointensity and STIR T2 hyperintensity owing to bone marrow edema resulting from a recent vertebral collapse that was causing pain (clinical correspondence). Normal signal intensity at the other lumbar vertebral bodies.

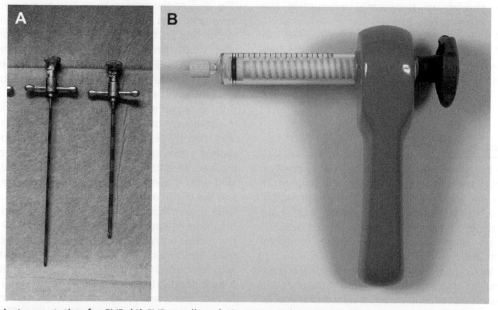

Fig. 2. Instrumentation for PVP. (*A*) PVP needles of 13 gauge and 11 gauge. (*B*) Cement injection kit.

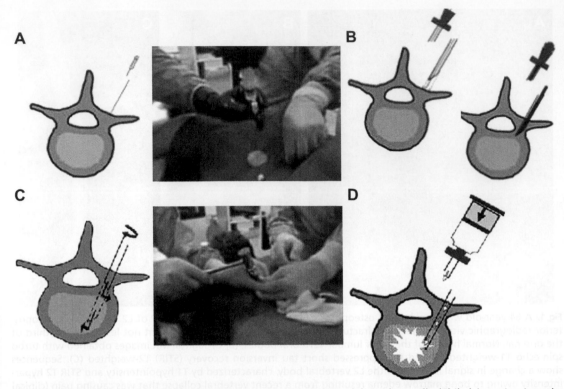

Fig. 3. Drawing of the main phases of percutaneous vertebroplasty. (*A*) Guide needle (Chiba) insertion into the periosteum and local anesthesia. (*B*) On the guide needle, coaxial introduction of the cannula (with bevelled distal end) and insertion into the bone cortex. After removal of the guide needle, the stylet is reinserted into the cannula and the needle enters the vertebral body through the pedicle. (*C*) The direction of needle penetration depends on the orientation of the bevel tip, obtained by rotating (*curved arrow*) the external portion of the needle. With the bevel tip oriented laterally, the needle avoids the spinal canal, whereas with the bevel tip oriented medially, the needle approaches the center of the body (*arrows*). (*D*) Once the needle is in place, the stylet is removed and the acrylic cement is slowly injected.

slowing or temporarily interrupting the injection (see **Fig. 4**B)

A floor pedal to control the scan (see **Fig. 4**B)

A control joystick to move the CT table (see **Fig. 4**C)

Software packages for real-time image display and radiation dose containment (Hand-CARE)

Procedure

Once the patient was placed in the prone position and was as comfortable as possible, a stack of CT scans was acquired to visualize the axial or sagittal and coronal MPR images. This procedure enabled us to choose the best anatomic approach depending on individual anatomy and vertebral alterations.[1]

At the dorsal level where the pedicles have a smaller diameter and limited obliquity, the approach was mainly parapedicular and unilateral transcostovertebral, across the articulation plane (**Fig. 5**).[2] At the lumbar level, where the pedicles have sufficient diameter and obliquity to reach the central portion of the vertebra, the approach was more frequently unilateral transpedicular than bilateral (**Fig. 6**).[3] The lateral approach was used only in few cases (11 PVPs) at the lumbar level following an oblique pathway.

In a single session, we treated from one to a maximum of four vertebrae. Targeting was achieved by placing a small metal chain on the patient's skin at the level of treatment to define the needle entry point (marked on the patient's skin with a surgical marking pen), the obliquity, and the depth of the needle pathway. The surgical field was prepared by sterilizing the skin over a surface of approximately 80 cm² and delimiting the needle entry point with large sterile drapes to minimize risks of infection. After local anesthesia with lidocaine hydrochloride (1%), the guide needle included in the kit or a Chiba needle was introduced percutaneously and advanced until it reached the vertebral periosteum (see **Fig. 3**A).

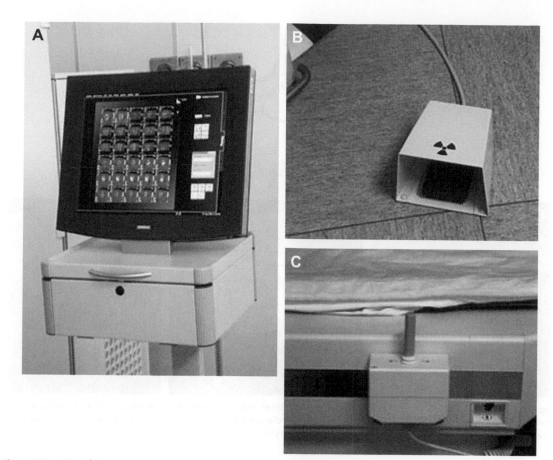

Fig. 4. CT-optional instrumentation for fluoroscopic control. (*A*) 17-in liquid-crystal monitor, (*B*) floor pedal, (*C*) control joystick.

At this stage, deep local anesthesia can be administered through the guide needle. The dose of anesthetic used was 2 to 3 mL for each vertebra, as suggested in the literature.[10] The maximum amount of lidocaine hydrochloride (1%) that can be administered is approximately 20 mL, as indicated in the guidelines of the Italian Pharmaceutical Agency.[11]

After performing a small incision in the skin with the scalpel and cutting the external tip of the Chiba needle, we used the needle as a guide to advance the PVP cannula without the stylet, coaxially, until it penetrated the cortical bone (see **Fig.** 3A, B). Before removing the Chiba needle, we always checked the correct position and obliquity of the cannula by CT. The stylet was then reinserted into the PVP cannula choosing the diamond tip for a linear advancement or, more often, the bevel tip to orient needle direction (see **Fig.** 3C). Needle advancement through the cortical and trabecular bone was achieved with the aid of the surgical hammer under fluoroscopic guidance in a lateral projection or with CT fluoroscopy in the axial plane. Once the needle was positioned in the

vertebral body, a biopsy was obtained with a core biopsy needle introduced coaxially into the PVP cannula but only when the initial diagnostic assessment had failed to identify the nature of the vertebral alteration (14 patients). Preparation and injection of the acrylic cement took a variable time depending on the number of vertebrae to treat. We generally prepare the cement after placement of the needle into the vertebra, because acrylic cement at ambient temperature maintains a suitable viscosity for injection no longer than 6 to 8 minutes. The optimal viscosity of acrylic cement is similar to that of toothpaste; in fact, insufficient viscosity increases the risk for cement leaks, whereas excessive viscosity may cause difficulty in injecting the cement and filling the vertebral body. In our experience, we never used ice-bath cooling to delay cement polymerization.[10–13] The amount of acrylic cement injected in each vertebra ranged from 2 mL to 9 mL (mean 5.7).

The injection monitoring was done under radiofluoroscopic guidance in 135 PVPs to check cement distribution in the vertebral body or identify

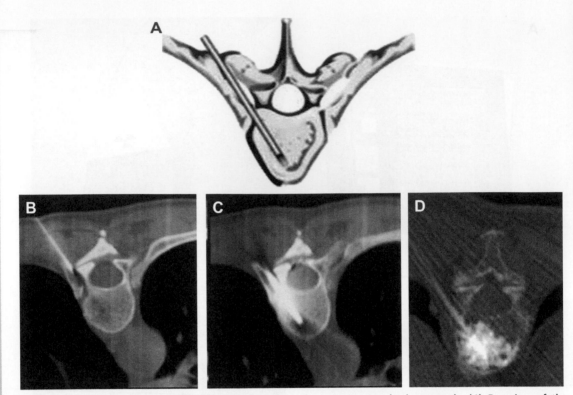

Fig. 5. Dorsal percutaneous vertebroplasty with unilateral transcostovertebral approach. (*A*) Drawing of the correct needle placing. (*B*) CT fluoroscopy–guided needle positioning. (*C*) CT fluoroscopy–guided PVP cannula positioning. (*D*) Fluoroscopy-guided injection of the acrylic cement.

possible leakages. In the remaining 47 PVPs, all steps, including cement injection, were monitored by axial CT fluoroscopy alone (see **Figs. 5**C and **6**B–D). The detection of a leak always required slowing or interrupting the injection. At the end of the injection, the stylet was reinserted to push the cement remaining in the cannula into the vertebral body. To avoid the risk for spreading the cement in the soft tissues,[3,10] approximately 10 minutes after the injection the needle was slowly removed by rotating and withdrawing it gently. After the procedure we obtained a series of CT scans to evaluate and document, in the axial, coronal, and sagittal planes, the intrasomatic distribution of the cement (see **Fig. 5**D), extent and extension of possible leaks (see **Fig. 6**C–E), and soft tissues hematomas. When pulmonary complications (acrylic cement embolus, pneumothorax, or hemothorax) were suspected, the CT study was extended to the chest (8 patients). After CT final assessment, patients were instructed to get off the table and maintain an upright position for about 1 minute to check their clinical condition immediately after PVP before transferring them to the ward. Patients lay in a supine position for about 3 hours after the procedure. Most patients were discharged from hospital within 24 hours

(104 patients); 2 patients remained in hospital for 3 days after the procedure because of severe complications requiring treatment and a period of observation.

Follow-up

The follow-up of the first 106 patients was performed by the internist. During the first follow-up visit, patients were administered the same questionnaire used for the preoperative assessment. During the follow-up, 67 of 106 patients underwent radiographic examination of the dorsolumbar spine regardless of clinical symptoms.

Evaluation of treatment outcome was done in all patients within 24 hours of the procedure and during the follow-up by comparing data of the questionnaires before and after PVP.

The clinical results were therefore based on the scales assessing pain, functional mobility, and analgesic use.

Complications were divided into mild (conditions requiring bland therapy or a 24-hour observation period in hospital) and severe (conditions requiring more aggressive treatment or hospitalization for more than 24 hours).

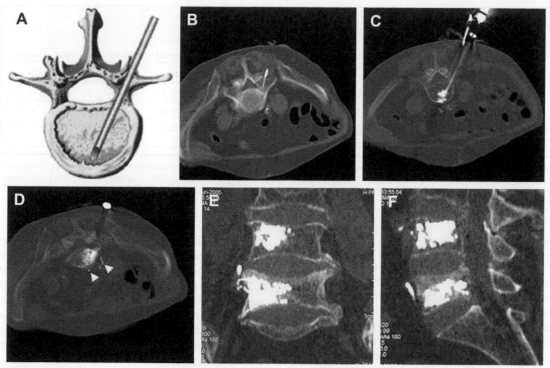

Fig. 6. Lumbar percutaneous vertebroplasty with unilateral transpedicular approach at the levels of L4 and L5 (osteoporotic fractures). (*A*) Drawing of the correct needle placing at L5. (*B*) CT-guided insertion of the PDP cannula. (*C*) Control during cement injection in the body. (*D*) During the injection, small venous anterior leakages of cement (*arrows*) are seen, without clinical symptoms. (*E*, *F*) Postprocedural CT scan: the sagittal and coronal images obtained with MPR demonstrate cement distribution with a small, cranially oriented, anterior venous leakage.

Extravertebral cement leakages were not considered complications unless they were accompanied by clinical symptoms; therefore, for the purposes of statistical analysis, all cement leakages, whether mild or severe, were classified according to their site: paravertebral, intradiscal, epidural, foraminal, and vascular. Recurrences were subdivided into osteoporotic vertebral collapse or metastases appearing in other dorso-lumbar vertebrae after PVP.

RESULTS

All the data relative to the first series of patients have been presented and discussed in a previous publication,[4] so we report only the most relevant results here.

We treated from one to a maximum of four vertebrae in a single session, with a mean value of 1.7 vertebrae/patient. Mean overall procedure time was 57.5 ± 20 minutes (range 21 minutes for one vertebra, 128 minutes for four); mean procedure time for the treatment of one vertebra was slightly longer in metastasis (35.5 minutes) than in osteoporotic collapses (31.6 minutes). With regard to clinical outcome, pain reduction within 24 hours of treatment was significant or complete in 104 patients (98%). The results of the assessment of pain, functional mobility, and analgesic use before and after PVP are summarized in **Table 1**.

Statistical analysis indicated a significant improvement ($P < .001$) in pain and analgesic use after PVP.

We had three severe complications (one pneumothorax and two symptomatic leakages) (2.8%) requiring treatment and a 3-day hospital stay after PVP. There were two mild complications (cement pulmonary embolism) (1.8%), requiring an observation period of 24 hours after PVP.

Structural collapse in vertebral bodies close to those treated with PVP were identified in eight cases (11.9%) in the group of patients receiving anti–bone-resorption agents; half of them were symptomatic. In neoplastic patients, the appearance of new symptomatic vertebral localizations after PVP was detected in two cases (5.1%), one at 4 months (kidney) and the other at 5.5 months (breast).

Table 1
Results of the clinical evaluation.

Clinical Evaluation	Score	Total Series (106 Patients)		Osteoporosis (67 Patients)		Metastases (39 Patients)	
		Pre-PVP	Post-PVP	Pre-PVP	Post-PVP	Pre-PVP	Post-PVP
Pain (VAS)	1–10	8.57 ± 0.61	2.80 ± 1.30	8.51 ± 0.53	2.78 ± 1.27	8.62 ± 0.71	2.84 ± 1.36
Mobility	1–4	3.10 ± 0.66	1.19 ± 0.54	3.10 ± 0.68	1.16 ± 0.48	3.25 ± 0.59	1.24 ± 0.64
Analgesic use	1–3	2.98 ± 0.19	1.16 ± 0.50	2.96 ± 0.24	1.12 ± 0.45	3.00	1.24 ± 0.59

Mean values with standard deviation of the three clinical evaluation score systems (visual analogue scale [VAS], functional mobility, analgesic use) observed before percutaneous vertebroplasty (pre-PVP) and after treatment (post-PVP) are shown for the whole series (106), for patients who had osteoporosis (67) and for those who had metastases (39).

DISCUSSION

Painful vertebral collapse is sometimes difficult to prevent and treat with simple conservative therapy and can become difficult to manage for pain reduction and vertebral body consolidation in patients who have osteoporosis or neoplasia. Following these indications, we predominantly treated osteoporotic vertebral collapses (63.2%), with fewer cases of cancer metastases (33%) or myeloma (3.8%). Among the selection criteria adopted, concordance of the clinical assessment (pain site) and imaging findings (structural alteration level) is the most important indication.[3,4,7] In particular, when selecting patients, MRI findings of bone marrow edema (see **Fig. 1**B, C) associated with pain should be considered a sign of recent vertebral involvement and therefore predictive of a positive response to PVP.[14–16] Imaging allowed us to verify the existence of anatomic compatibility for the PVP procedure by excluding the following clinical conditions:[17]

> Severe vertebral collapse (height less than one third of original height),
> Posterior wall or pedicle involvement,
> Spinal cord compression
> Osteosclerosis of the vertebral trabecular network.

The first 135 PVPs (74%) were performed with CT in combination with radiofluoroscopy, because this was believed to be safer and more precise compared with radiofluoroscopic guidance alone. Subsequently, after our department acquired a multislice CT scanner equipped with fluoroscopic capabilities, the remaining 47 PVPs (26%) were performed under CT guidance alone. The use of CT with or without radiofluoroscopy allows an easier targeting of the vertebral body and enables a multiplanar evaluation of the vertebra before and after PVP;[18–22] it is thus preferred to

other techniques. The preferred needle routes were transpedicular (61%) for the lumbar level and transcostovertebral (30.7%) for the dorsal level. CT fluoroscopy facilitates evaluation of cement distribution, allowing immediate detection of leakages in any direction on the axial views (see **Fig. 6**C, D). Because there is no correlation between the amount of acrylic cement injected and symptom remission,[4,10,17] we tried to achieve a good central distribution of cement within the vertebral body.

A single level session lasted an average time of 57 minutes, with a mean time per vertebra only slightly longer for metastases compared with osteoporotic collapses; this has been well tolerated by all our patients without any anesthesiologic support.

Pain reduction was recorded in 98% of patients within 24 hours of the treatment.

In literature studies on the treatment of metastases, pain disappearance or reduction was reported in 75% to 82% of patients,[23–25] whereas in the treatment of osteoporotic collapse it was reported in 73% to 97%.[7,8,26–28] In mixed series including both metastases and osteoporosis (more similar to our series) pain disappearance or reduction was reported in 75% to 100% of cases within 1 week.[3,25,29–35] Reduction in analgesic use and improvement in functional mobility observed in our study confirmed that PVP had an overall positive effect on quality of life, with a possible reduction of health care costs. If patient selection is accurate and the procedure is performed following a meticulous technique, complications are rare[36,37] and more common in metastases (5%) than in osteoporotic collapse (1%). In our experience, CT guidance helped to limit the incidence of severe (2.8%) and mild (1.8%) complications reported in other studies.[17,33–35,37,38] Infections are avoided by antibiotic prophylaxis in immunocompromised patients, accurate sterilization of the surgical field, and a rigorous aseptic technique.[14,17,37] As reported in the literature,[39-42] fracture recurrences within 1 year after PVP are frequent in patients who have osteoporosis (12.4%–21.7%) supported by the relationship between the treated vertebral body and the adjacent ones, osteoporosis progression, and increased mobility. We found a fracture recurrence rate of 11.9% in osteoporotic patients and new symptomatic vertebral metastases in 5.1% in oncology patients; most recurrences occurred within 1 year after the treatment.

In conclusion, our experience suggests that patient selection should be preferably carried out by a multidisciplinary team to ensure an optimal level of accuracy that only the combination of specialist competence in the clinical and imaging fields can guarantee. The use of a CT-guided technique to perform PVP procedures enhances safety and precision of the targeting in cement injection operations, thereby reducing the risk for complications. This finding is particularly important when a team embarks on an experience with this procedure and needs to minimize the risks and problems related to the learning curve. For this reason we think that performing PVP in a radiology department equipped with the best image-guiding technology (radiofluoroscopy or CT), where the competence of other specialists and the radiologist can come together, represents the optimal solution to ensure the best chances of success and reduce the risk for complications.

SUMMARY

The use of percutaneous vertebroplasty (PVP) is a minimally invasive option in the treatment of osteoporotic or metastatic vertebral collapses. Our personal experience, using a CT-guided technique, confirms the efficacy and safety of PVP with a lower risk for complications compared with conventional fluoroscopic approaches because of a precise placement of the instruments in the vertebral body and an early detection of small cement leakages.

Partial or complete pain relief was obtained in 98% of patients within 24 hours of the treatment; significant results were also obtained regarding improvement in functional mobility and reduction of analgesic use. Severe complications were one case of pneumothorax and two cases of symptomatic cement leakage. Mild complications included two cases of cement pulmonary embolism; all recovered without any procedure. During the follow-up, eight patients who had osteoporosis presented a new vertebral fracture (12%), and new

vertebral metastases appeared in two oncologic patients (5%).

REFERENCES

1. Galibert P, Deramond H, Rosat P, et al. Preliminary note on the treatment of vertebral angioma by percutaneous acrylic vertebroplasty. Neurochirurgie 1987; 33:166–8.

2. Jensen ME, Evans AJ, Mathis JM, et al. Percutaneous polymethyl-methacrylate vertebroplasty in the treatment of osteoporotic vertebral body compression fractures: technical aspects. AJNR Am J Neuroradiol 1997;18:1897–904.

3. Hide IG, Gangi A. Percutaneous vertebroplasty: history, technique and current perspectives. Clin Radiol 2004;59:461–7.

4. Caudana R, Renzi Brivio L, Ventura L, et al. CT-guided percutaneous vertebroplasty: personal experience in the treatment of osteoporotic fractures and dorsolumbar metastases. Radiol Med 2008;113: 114–33.

5. Barr JD, Mathis JM, Barr MS, et al. Standard for the performance of percutaneous vertebroplasty. In: American College of Radiology standards [ACR] 2000–2001. Reston (VA): ACR; 2000. p. 339–45.

6. McCaffery M, Pasero C. Visual analogic scale [VAS]. In: McCaffery M, Pasero C, editors. Pain: clinical manual. St Louis (MO): Mosby; 1999. p. 6.

7. Zoarsky GH, Snow P, Olan WJ, et al. Percutaneous vertebroplasty for osteoporotic compression fractures: quantitative prospective evaluation of long-term outcomes. J Vasc Interv Radiol 2002;13: 139–48.

8. Peh WC, Gilula LA, Peck DD. Percutaneous vertebroplasty for severe osteoporotic vertebral body compression fractures. Radiology 2002;223:121–6.

9. Kirby BS, Doyle A, Gilula LA. Acute bronchospasm due to exposure to polymethylmethacrylate vapors during percutaneous vertebroplasty. AJR Am J Roentgenol 2003;180:543–4.

10. Mathis JM, Wong W. Percutaneous vertebroplasty: technical considerations. J Vasc Interv Radiol 2003;14:953–60.

11. Agenzia Italiana del Farmaco [AIFA]. Lidocaina. In: Masson, editor. Guida all'uso dei farmaci 3. Milano (MI): Masson; 2005. p. 1935.

12. Chavali R, Resijek R, Knight SK, et al. Extending polymerization time of polymethylmethacrylate cement in percutaneous vertebroplasty with ice bath cooling. AJNR Am J Neuroradiol 2003;24: 545–6.

13. Weill A, Chiras J, Simon JM, et al. Spinal metastases: indications for and results of percutaneous injection of acrylic surgical cement. Radiology 1996;199:241–7.

14. Mathis JM, Barr JD, Belkoff SM, et al. Percutaneous vertebroplasty: a developing standard of care for vertebral compression fractures. AJNR Am J Neuroradiol 2001;22:373–81.

15. Tanigawa N, Komemushi A, Kariya S, et al. Percutaneous vertebroplasty: relationship between vertebral body bone marrow edema pattern on MR images and initial clinical response. Radiology 2006;239:195–200.

16. Brown DB, Glaiberman CB, Gilula LA, et al. Correlation between preprocedural MRI findings and clinical outcomes in the treatment of chronic symptomatic vertebral compression fractures with percutaneous vertebroplasty. AJR Am J Roentgenol 2005;184:1951–5.

17. Cotten A, Boutry N, Cortet B, et al. Percutaneous vertebroplasty: state of the art. Radiographics 1998;18:311–20.

18. Katada K, Kato R, Anno H, et al. Guidance with real-time CT fluoroscopy: early clinical experience. Radiology 1996;200:851–6.

19. Carlson SK, Bender CE, Classic KL, et al. Benefits and safety of CT fluoroscopy in interventional radiologic procedures. Radiology 2001;219:515–20.

20. Weber CH, Krotz M, Hoffmann RT, et al. CT-guided vertebroplasty and kyphoplasty: comparing technical success rate and complications in 101cases. Rofo 2006;178:610–7.

21. Kim JH, Park KS, Yi S, et al. Real-time CT fluoroscopy (CTF)-guided vertebroplasty in osteoporotic spine fractures. Yonsei Med J 2005;46:635–42.

22. Deramond H, Depriester C, Galibert P, et al. Percutaneous vertebroplasty with polymethylmethacrylate. Technique, indications, and results. Radiol Clin North Am 1998;36:533–46.

23. Shimony JS, Gilula LA, Zeller AJ, et al. Percutaneous vertebroplasty for malignant compression fractures with epidural involvement. Radiology 2004;232: 846–53.

24. Martin JB, Wetzel SG, Seium Y, et al. Percutaneous vertebroplasty in metastatic disease: transpedicular access and treatment of lysed pedicles—initial experience. Radiology 2003;229:593–7.

25. Fourney DR, Schomer DF, Nader R, et al. Percutaneous vertebroplasty and kyphoplasty for painful vertebral body fractures in cancer patients. J Neurosurg 2003;98:21–30.

26. Gangi A, Kastler BA, Dietemann JL. Percutaneous vertebroplasty guided by a combination of CT and fluoroscopy. AJNR Am J Neuroradiol 1994;15:83–6.

27. Kim AK, Jensen ME, Dion JE, et al. Unilateral transpedicular percutaneous vertebroplasty: initial experience. Radiology 2002;222:737–41.

28. Molloy S, Riley LH 3rd, Belkoff SM. Effect of cement volume and placement on mechanical-property restoration resulting fromvertebroplasty. AJNR Am J Neuroradiol 2005;26:401–4.

29. Cotten A, Dewatre F, Cortet B, et al. Percutaneous vertebroplasty for osteolytic metastases and myeloma: effects of the percentage of lesion filling and the leakage of methylmethacrylate at clinical follow-up. Radiology 1996;200:525–30.

30. Dublin AB, Hartman J, Latchaw RE, et al. The vertebral body fracture in osteoporosis: restoration of height using percutaneous vertebroplasty. AJNR Am J Neuroradiol 2005;26:489–92.

31. Gangi A, Guth S, Imbert JP, et al. Percutaneous vertebroplasty: indications, technique, and results. Radiographics 2003;23:10–20.

32. Barr JD, Barr MS, Lemley TJ, et al. Percutaneous vertebroplasty for pain relief and spinal stabilization. Spine 2000;25:923–8.

33. Muto M, Muto E, Izzo R, et al. Vertebroplasty in the treatment of back pain. Radiol Med 2005;109:208–19.

34. Hodler J, Peck D, Gilula LA. Midterm outcome after vertebroplasty: predictive value of technical and patient-related factors. Radiology 2003;227:662–8.

35. Anselmetti GC, Corgnier A, Debernardi F, et al. Treatment of painful compression vertebral fractures with vertebroplasty: results and complications. Radiol Med 2005;110:262–72.

36. Mousavi P, Roth S, Finkelstein J, et al. Volumetric quantification of cement leakage following percutaneous vertebroplasty in metastatic and osteoporotic vertebrae. J Neurosurg 2003;99(Suppl 1):56–9.

37. Mathis JM. Percutaneous vertebroplasty: complication avoidance and technique optimization. AJNR Am J Neuroradiol 2003;24:1697–706.

38. Padovani B, Kasriel O, Brunner P, et al. Pulmonary embolism caused by acrylic cement: a rare complication of percutaneous vertebroplasty. AJNR Am J Neuroradiol 1999;20:375–7.

39. Verlaan JJ, Oner FC, Slootweg PJ, et al. Histologic changes after vertebroplasty. J Bone Joint Surg Am 2004;86:1230–8.

40. Baroud G, Nemes J, Heini P, et al. Load shift of the intervertebral disc after a vertebroplasty: a finite-element study. Eur Spine J 2003;12:421–6.

41. Uppin AA, Hirsch JA, Centenera LV, et al. Occurrence of new vertebral body fracture after percutaneous vertebroplasty in patients with osteoporosis. Radiology 2003;226:119–24.

42. Syed MI, Patel NA, Jan S, et al. New symptomatic vertebral compression fractures within a year following vertebroplasty in osteoporotic women. Spine 2005;26:1601–4.

Thoracoscopy for Minimally Invasive Thoracic Spine Surgery

Umile Giuseppe Longo, MD[a], Nicola Papapietro, MD[a],
Nicola Maffulli, MD, MS, PhD, FRCS (Orth)[b],*, Vincenzo Denaro, MD[a]

KEYWORDS

- Thoracoscopy • Minimally invasive surgery
- Spine • Tumors • Osteoid osteoma
- Video-assisted thoracic surgery

Thoracoscopy, first performed by Cruise in Dublin in 1865,[1] was popularized in Stockholm in the first decades of the twentieth century by Jacobaeus, an internist who is still regarded as the father of thoracoscopy.[2] Thoracoscopy has been used worldwide for many years by thoracic surgeons for the diagnosis and management of lysis of pleural adhesions, tuberculous and malignant effusions, and varies lung pathologic conditions.[3] Recent advances in thoracoscopy and a new trend toward minimally invasive procedures have brought surgeons to coin the term "surgical" thoracoscopy, or video-assisted thoracic surgery (VATS).[4–6] The term "medical thoracoscopy" appeared approximately 20 years ago with the introduction of VATS to differentiate it from the old conventional thoracoscopy technique described by Jacobaeus.[2] VATS gained a well-deserved place in the thoracic surgeon armamentarium.[7] It has altered the standard of practice in the management of diseases of the chest wall, pleura, and esophagus. To date, it is gaining a space in orthopedic practice, taking advantage of the experience of other specialties.[8] In the orthopedic field, VATS has been used successfully in anterior thoracic and thoracolumbar spine surgery.[9–11] Obenchain first performed a lumbar disc resection through laparoscopy in 1991.[12] In 1994, Rosenthal described a technique of microsurgical endoscopy for removal of protruded thoracic discs.[13]

Despite a long learning curve and the technical demands of the procedure, VATS has several advantages, including better cosmesis, adequate exposure to all levels of the thoracic spine from T2 to L1, better illumination and magnification at the site of surgery, less damage to the tissue adjacent to the surgical field, less morbidity when compared with standard thoracotomy in terms of respiratory problems, pain, blood loss, and muscle and chest wall damages, consequent shorter recovery time, less postoperative pulmonary function impairment, and shorter hospitalization.[1,14–19] Advantages for surgeons include a magnified view of the surgical field, adequate management of bleeding vessels because of better identification and less perioperative blood loss, and adequate anterior magnification of the dural sac and origin of nerve roots.[20,21] A thoracic surgeon familiar with thoracoscopy and standard thoracotomy should be available to assist during the procedure, especially at the beginning of the learning curve.[22] The anesthesiologist must be familiar with the use of double-lumen tubes with one-lung ventilation. Specialized equipment is required for VATS, including telescopes, light sources, cameras, monitors, and appropriate instrumentation.[23–25]

The aim of this article is to describe the state-of-the-art of thoracoscopy in the diagnosis and management of common thoracic spine orthopedic conditions.

The authors declare no conflict of interest. No funding was received for this study.

[a] Department of Orthopaedic and Trauma Surgery, Campus Biomedico University, Via Alvaro Del Portillo, 200, 00128 Trigoria, Rome, Italy

[b] Centre for Sports and Exercise Medicine Queen Mary University of London, Barts and The London School of Medicine and Dentistry, Mile End Hospital, 275 Bancroft Road, London E1 4DG, UK

* Corresponding author.
E-mail address: n.maffulli@qmul.ac.uk (N. Maffulli).

Orthop Clin N Am 40 (2009) 459–464
doi:10.1016/j.ocl.2009.05.005
0030-5898/09/$ – see front matter © 2009 Elsevier Inc. All rights reserved.

INDICATIONS

Indications for VATS apparently are the same as those for standard thoracotomy. Extensive internal fixation can be difficult to perform during VATS, however.[6,26–28] In such instances, an open approach may be required, and patients should provide consent to convert VATS to standard thoracotomy if necessary.[15] VATS is currently being used in the spine when an anterior approach is indicated. Indications for VATS in the thoracic spine include scoliosis, Scheuermann's disease, hemivertebrae, crankshaft deformities, tumor resections, spinal decompression in fractures, decompression of nerve roots in degenerative processes, and correction of thoracic deformities.[27,29] Contraindications to performing VATS are the inability to tolerate single-lung ventilation, high airway pressures with positive pressure ventilation, emphysema, severe or acute respiratory insufficiency, and previous thoracotomy.[15]

TECHNIQUE

Patients undergo general anesthesia with either a double-lumen endotracheal tube or a bronchial blocker for single-lung ventilation to obtain a selective collapse of the lung on the involved side.[7,30,31] Before starting the procedure, the anesthesiologist is required to deflate the lung. Patients are placed in a lateral decubitus position on a radiolucent operating table to allow radiographic control. The right-sided approach is recommended unless technical contraindications are present. Two pillows—on the ventral and dorsal sides— attached to the table are used to pad the patient. The legs are well supported with a pillow between them. All the bony prominences are padded to avoid compression. The upper arm is placed on a stand with the shoulder slightly abducted and flexed over 90°. In some patients, it is useful to put a pillow under the thoracic region of the patient to elevate the thoracic spine and open the intervertebral spaces to prevent the risk of neurologic damage.[4,29,32]

Generally the surgeon stands on the anterior side of the patient's thorax to have a frontal view of the spine. The first assistant stands to the left of the surgeon, and the second assistant stands in front of them on the posterior side of the thorax.[7] This positioning of the surgeons allows more space for the monitors and all the surgical instruments. The number, position, and size of the portals vary according to the choice of the surgeon and location of the lesion to be addressed.[7] The trocar is commonly placed in the seventh or eighth intercostal space at level of the posterior axillary

line. The first one is the only portal positioned without visual control, and caution is needed. The incision is performed over the top of the rib to avoid damage to the intercostal vessels and nerves. The other incisions can be performed in the intercostal spaces corresponding to the anterior axillary line according to the level of the problem. During VATS, the thoracic spine can be divided into three regions (T1-5, T6-9, and T10-L1) with peculiar anatomy. A 30° angled telescope is inserted through the trocar. The viewing port is placed in the posterior axillary line, and two or three working ports are commonly placed in the anterior axillary line. The portals can be placed cephalad or caudad, depending on the level of the thoracic spine to be reached. The patient is placed in a reverse Trendelenburg position to approach the upper thoracic spine or Trendelenburg position to approach the lower thoracic spine. When completely collapsed, the lung normally falls away from the surgical field.[4,29,32,33]

A diagnostic thoracoscopy is performed to determine the spinal level to which surgery must be performed. Ribs attach to vertebrae via costotransverse and costovertebral ligaments. The rib heads articulate with the base of the pedicle and the vertebral body just below disk or at disk space and are important landmarks for location of the level. The confirmation of the level at which the surgery must be performed is important, because surgery can be performed at the wrong level if an incorrect vertebral count is done. A check film with a metal marker is mandatory.[34–37]

The parietal pleura are sectioned with the monopolar cautery to free all soft tissues. In patients in whom extension of lower exposure is required, the diaphragm can be opened. Preservation of the vessels located over the vertebral bodies is highly recommended, because it can be difficult to control bleeding endoscopically. All the vessels that seem to be at risk for bleeding should be coagulated. Through blunt dissection in correspondence with the anterolateral side of the disc, the longitudinal anterior ligament is exposed. With the monopolar cautery, the annulus fibrosus is incised to prepare a window through which the content of the intervertebral disc is extracted.[5,13,38] Hemostatic products can be useful for controlling bleeding from the disc space.[7] A corpectomy is usually performed after discectomy at the adjacent levels of the involved vertebra and successive removal of the vertebral body until the posterior longitudinal ligament is reached. Reconstruction and stabilization can be performed in several ways, depending on the size, location, and preferences of the surgeon.[7]

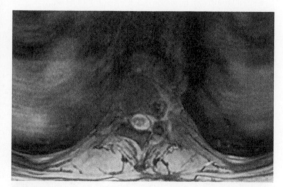

Fig. 1. MRI axial view of the thoracic spine of a patient shows the presence of a nidus with a sclerotic rim in the body of the tenth thoracic vertebra.

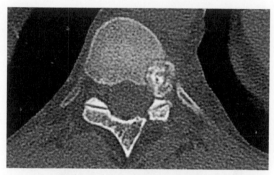

Fig. 3. CT axial view of the thoracic spine of a patient shows the presence of a nidus with a sclerotic rim in the body of the tenth thoracic vertebra.

A chest tube must be inserted at the end of surgery through the most posterior inferior portal. The endoscope must be used to observe the chest tube, and the tube must be connected to a water seal. After the anesthesiologist has inflated the lung to determine if air leaks exist, the portals are closed in routine fashion. Postoperatively, patients usually complain of minimal pain, and ventilatory function is not compromised. Patients remain in bed and follow an inhalotherapeutic program. Walking or sitting is allowed 24 hours after surgery.

PITFALLS AND COMPLICATIONS

Pitfalls and complications of VATS for thoracic spine surgery are the same as those that occur during open procedures. They include pitfalls of diagnosis, complications related to anesthesiologic problems, complications related to patient positioning, complications involving surgical approaches, complications related to the specific pathologic condition, complications related to bone graft, wrong level surgery, and pitfalls related

to inadequate or incomplete surgical technique or inadequate spinal immobilization.[7] The most common specific pitfalls of VATS include atelectasis, prolonged air leak, hemorrhage, and infection. Persistent atelectasis may lead to hypoxia and pneumonia. Patients require aggressive pulmonary toilet (ambulation, bronchodilators, and coughing) to obtain resolution. Specific complications of thoracoscopy include trocar injuries and intercostal neuritis.[7,34]

Every organ in the hemithorax can be damaged with blind trocar placement. The best way to prevent trocar injuries is to place the first port under direct vision, with others placed under thoracoscopic guidance.[34] It can be difficult to control bleeding endoscopically. All vessels that seem to be at risk for bleeding should be coagulated. A radiopaque sponge should be available at all times to apply pressure. After application of direct pressure, electrocautery should be used for hemostasis. Endoscopic clip appliers or other hemostatic agents must be available during surgery.[34] Damage to the lung may occur during VATS. Air leak may be repaired with an endoscopic stapler. Dural tears also may occur and must be

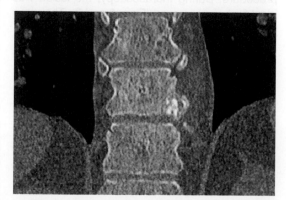

Fig. 2. CT coronal view of the thoracic spine of a patient shows the presence of a nidus with a sclerotic rim in the body of the tenth thoracic vertebra.

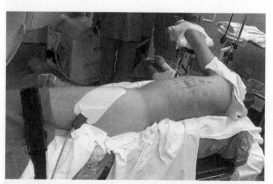

Fig. 4. Patient was placed in a lateral decubitus position.

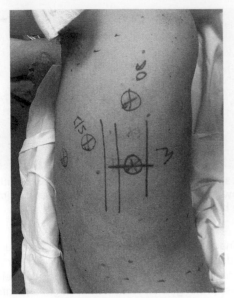

Fig. 5. A detail of positioning of portals.

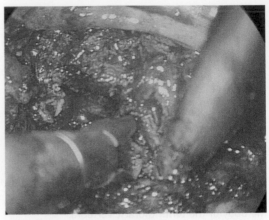

Fig. 7. The lesion was removed.

recognized and managed immediately. Small leakage of clear cerebrospinal fluid can be managed with hemostatic agents. Larger leakage of clear cerebrospinal fluid requires thoracotomy and vertebrectomy with dural repair.[13,36,37]

Lymphatic injury may be closed with an endoscopic clip applier. Damage to the thoracic duct also may occur, especially at the level of the diaphragm. Chylothorax diagnosed postoperatively is managed with a low-fat diet.[34] Damage to the sympathetic nerve chain on the operative side causes little or no morbidity. Consequences of sympathetic nerve chain damage include temperature and skin color changes below the level of the surgery. Postoperative pulmonary problems often involve the downside lung, in which mucous plugs

can form. The anesthesiologist should suction both lungs before extubation.[15]

ILLUSTRATIVE CASE REPORT

In September 2008, a 27-year-old man complained of persistent thoracic spine pain. The onset of the symptoms was light pain that became worse at night and limited the patient's daily activities. The use of aspirin typically helped to alleviate the pain. Laboratory test results were within normal range. Radiographs showed no remarkable findings. MRI (Fig. 1) and CT (Figs. 2 and 3) scans of his thoracic spine revealed the presence of a nidus with a sclerotic rim in the body of the tenth thoracic vertebra. Bone scan showed increased uptake corresponding to the lesion. The patient underwent thoracoscopy. The patient was placed in a lateral decubitus position (Fig. 4). A detail of position of portals is presented in Fig. 5. Prophylactic antibiotics were given for 24 hours, beginning at initiation of the surgical procedure. During thoracoscopy, the lesion was identified and removed (Figs. 6 and 7). The mass

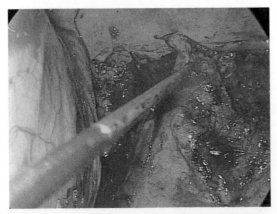

Fig. 6. The confirmation of the level was performed.

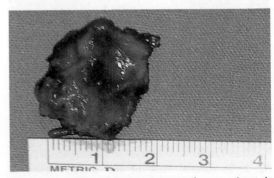

Fig. 8. The removed lesion measured approximately 18 mm × 20 mm.

measured approximately 18 mm × 20 mm (**Fig. 8**). No other pathology was found in the chest. The gross bone specimen confirmed the presupposed diagnosis of osteoid osteoma. When last reviewed, the patient was symptom free.

SUMMARY

VATS is a promising technique with good results at short- and medium-term follow-up. It has several advantages over conventional thoracotomy. Appropriate selection of patients remains most important for determining a good postoperative outcome. Further studies are required to clarify the role of VATS in the management of thoracic spine pathologic conditions.

REFERENCES

1. Cruise FR. The endoscope as an aid to the diagnosis and treatment of disease. Br Med J 1865;8: 345–7.

2. Jacobeus HC. Über die möglichkeit die zystoskope bei untersuchung seroser hohlungen anzuwenden [Possibility of the use of cystoscope for investigation of serious cavities]. Munch Med Wochenschr 1910; 40:2090–2 [in German].

3. Jacobaeus HC. The cauterization of adhesions in artificial pneumothorax therapy of tuberculosis. Am Rev Tuberc 1922;6:871–97.

4. Miller JI Jr. Therapeutic thoracoscopy: new horizons for an established procedure. Ann Thorac Surg 1991;52(5):1036–7.

5. Santillan-Doherty P. [Video-assisted surgery in the management of thoracic problems]. Rev Invest Clin 1995;47(5):393–8 [in Spanish].

6. Loddenkemper R. Thoracoscopy: state of the art. Eur Respir J 1998;11(1):213–21.

7. McCullen GM, Criscitiello AA, Yuan HA. Principles of endoscopic techniques to the thoracic and lumbar spine. In: Mayer HM, editor. Minimally invasive spine surgery. Berlin: Springer-Verlag; 2006. p. 149–56.

8. Allan IJ, Vrana B, Greenwood R, et al. A "toolbox" for biological and chemical monitoring requirements for the European Union's Water Framework Directive. Talanta 2006;69(2):302–22.

9. Anand N, Regan JJ. Video-assisted thoracoscopic surgery for thoracic disc disease: classification and outcome study of 100 consecutive cases with a 2-year minimum follow-up period. Spine 2002; 27(8):871–9.

10. Assaker R, Cinquin P, Cotten A, et al. Image-guided endoscopic spine surgery: Part I. A feasibility study. Spine 2001;26(15):1705–10.

11. Bergey DL, Villavicencio AT, Goldstein T, et al. Endoscopic lateral transpsoas approach to the lumbar spine. Spine 2004;29(15):1681–8.

12. Obenchain TG. Laparoscopic lumbar discectomy: case report. J Laparoendosc Surg 1991;1(3):145–9.

13. Rosenthal D, Rosenthal R, de Simone A. Removal of a protruded thoracic disc using microsurgical endoscopy: a new technique. Spine 1994;19(9):1087–91.

14. Brody F, Rosen M, Tarnoff M, et al. Laparoscopic lateral L4-L5 disc exposure. Surg Endosc 2002; 16(4):650–3.

15. Canale ST. Campbell's operative orthopaedics. 10th edition. Philadelphia: Mosby; 2003.

16. Casey KF, Chang MK, O'Brien ED, et al. Arthroscopic microdiscectomy: comparison of preoperative and postoperative imaging studies. Arthroscopy 1997;13(4):438–45.

17. Dickman CA, Detweiler PW, Porter RW. Endoscopic spine surgery. Clin Neurosurg 2000;46:526–53.

18. Escobar E, Transfeldt E, Garvey T, et al. Video-assisted versus open anterior lumbar spine fusion surgery: a comparison of four techniques and complications in 135 patients. Spine 2003;28(7):729–32.

19. Guingrich JA, McDermott JC. Ureteral injury during laparoscopy-assisted anterior lumbar fusion. Spine 2000;25(12):1586–8.

20. Huang EY, Acosta JM, Gardocki RJ, et al. Thoracoscopic anterior spinal release and fusion: evolution of a faster, improved approach. J Pediatr Surg 2002;37(12):1732–5.

21. Huntington CF, Murrell WD, Betz RR, et al. Comparison of thoracoscopic and open thoracic discectomy in a live ovine model for anterior spinal fusion. Spine 1998;23(15):1699–702.

22. Kaiser MG, Haid RW Jr, Subach BR, et al. Comparison of the mini-open versus laparoscopic approach for anterior lumbar interbody fusion: a retrospective review. Neurosurgery 2002;51(1):97–103 [discussion: 103–5].

23. Kambin P, O'Brien E, Zhou L, et al. Arthroscopic microdiscectomy and selective fragmentectomy. Clin Orthop Relat Res 1998;347:150–67.

24. Kambin P, Zhou L. Arthroscopic dicoootomy of the lumbar spine. Clin Orthop Relat Res 1997;337: 49–57.

25. Khoo LT, Fessler RG. Microendoscopic decompressive laminotomy for the treatment of lumbar stenosis. Neurosurgery 2002;51(5 Suppl):S146–54.

26. Kleeman TJ, Michael Ahn U, Clutterbuck WB, et al. Laparoscopic anterior lumbar interbody fusion at L4-L5: an anatomic evaluation and approach classification. Spine 2002;27(13):1390–5.

27. Landreneau RJ, Mack MJ, Keenan RJ, et al. Strategic planning for video-assisted thoracic surgery. Ann Thorac Surg 1993;56(3):615–9.

28. Lieberman IH, Salo PT, Orr RD, et al. Prone position endoscopic transthoracic release with simultaneous posterior instrumentation for spinal deformity: a description of the technique. Spine 2000;25(17): 2251–7.

29. Moe JH. Modern concepts of treatment of spinal deformities in children and adults. Clin Orthop Relat Res 1980;150:137–53.

30. Mack MJ, Regan JJ, McAfee PC, et al. Video-assisted thoracic surgery for the anterior approach to the thoracic spine. Ann Thorac Surg 1995;59(5):1100–6.

31. McAfee PC, Regan JR, Zdeblick T, et al. The incidence of complications in endoscopic anterior thoracolumbar spinal reconstructive surgery: a prospective multicenter study comprising the first 100 consecutive cases. Spine 1995;20(14):1624–32.

32. Newton PO, Marks M, Faro F, et al. Use of video-assisted thoracoscopic surgery to reduce perioperative morbidity in scoliosis surgery. Spine 2003;28(20):S249–54.

33. Newton PO, Shea KG, Granlund KF. Defining the pediatric spinal thoracoscopy learning curve: sixty-five consecutive cases. Spine 2000;25(8):1028–35.

34. Ofluoglu O. Minimally invasive management of spinal metastases. Orthop Clin North Am 2009;40(1):155–68, viii.

35. Palmer S, Turner R, Palmer R. Bilateral decompressive surgery in lumbar spinal stenosis associated with spondylolisthesis: unilateral approach and use of a microscope and tubular retractor system [case series study]. Neurosurg Focus 2002;13(1):E4.

36. Regan JJ, Mack MJ, Picetti GD 3rd. A technical report on video-assisted thoracoscopy in thoracic spinal surgery: preliminary description. Spine 1995;20(7):831–7.

37. Regan JJ, Yuan H, McAfee PC. Laparoscopic fusion of the lumbar spine: minimally invasive spine surgery. A prospective multicenter study evaluating open and laparoscopic lumbar fusion. Spine 1999;24(4):402–11.

38. Ruetten S, Meyer O, Godolias G. Endoscopic surgery of the lumbar epidural space (epiduroscopy): results of therapeutic intervention in 93 patients. Minim Invasive Neurosurg 2003;46(1):1–4.

Vertebroplasty and Kyphoplasty: Reasons for Concern?

Luca Denaro, MD, PhD[a], Umile Giuseppe Longo, MD[b],*,
Vincenzo Denaro, MD[b]

KEYWORDS

- Vertebroplasty • Kyphoplasty • Vertebral body
- Vertebra • Fracture • Cementoplasty

Vertebral body fractures are a major health care problem in Western countries. They are a common cause of severe, debilitating pain with consequent reduced physical function. Pain and progressive loss of posture are the major problems related to these fractures, with an enormous impact on quality of life.[1,2]

Conservative management, including analgesics, bedrest, external fixation, and rehabilitation, is indicated in patients who do not have neurologic impairment. However, conservative management measures are only partially effective in symptom relief, and about one third of patients complain of persistent pain and progressive functional limitation and loss of mobility.[3] Moreover, antiinflammatory drugs are sometimes poorly tolerated by older patients, and bedrest can lead to further demineralization of the vertebrae, predisposing the patient to future fractures. Also, conservative management cannot prevent kyphotic deformity.

Surgery is indicated in patients who have symptoms refractory to conservative management modalities, and in patients who have concurrent spinal instability or neurologic deficit.[4,5] Open surgery can be difficult in older patients due to the poor quality of osteoporotic bone and age-related risks.

Two different minimally invasive percutaneous vertebral augmentation methods for cement application into the vertebral body to manage symptomatic compression fractures without neurologic impairment have been developed, namely, vertebroplasty and kyphoplasty.

In vertebroplasty, first reported in the literature in 1987 for the management of a painful, aggressive hemangioma of a vertebral body,[6] polymethylmethacrylate (PMMA) cement is injected percutaneously, under imaging guidance, into a collapsed vertebral body to strengthen it.

Kyphoplasty was introduced to manage the kyphotic deformity and help to realign the spine.[7] Kyphoplasty involves placing an inflatable bone tamp percutaneously into a vertebral body. The inflation of the bone tamp with fluid allows restoration of vertebral height and correction of kyphosis. After deflation, the cavity that has been produced is filled by injection of PMMA.

Kyphoplasty and vertebroplasty have gained wide acceptance in the treatment of patients who do not have neurologic impairment, and who have been suffering with otherwise unmanageable pain caused by vertebral compression fractures secondary to osteoporosis[8–10] or osteolytic changes[11] within a vertebral body. Both procedures depend on mechanical stabilization of the fracture produced by PMMA cement injection into the fractured vertebra.[12–15]

The exact mechanism of the analgesic effect of vertebral augmentation remains under debate. Pain reduction from the use of these percutaneous vertebral augmentation techniques has been attributed to the mechanical effects of the reconstruction and stabilization of the endplates and vertebral body segment by the stiffening of the cement, and to the therapeutic effect of the

[a] Department of Neurosurgery, Catholic University School of Medicine, Policlinico Gemelli, Largo Gemelli 8, 00168 Rome, Italy
[b] Department of Orthopaedic and Trauma Surgery, Campus Biomedico University, Via Alvaro del Portillo, 200, 00128 Rome, Italy
* Corresponding author.
E-mail address: g.longo@unicampus.it (U.G. Longo).

Orthop Clin N Am 40 (2009) 465–471
doi:10.1016/j.ocl.2009.05.004
0030-5898/09/$ – see front matter © 2009 Elsevier Inc. All rights reserved.

exothermic reaction of the cement, assuming that the pain originates from intraosseous nerve endings.[16] Despite widespread acceptance, some controversy remains regarding kyphoplasty and vertebroplasty, mainly with respect to height restoration, its clinical significance and the inherent risks thereof.[3,17–19]

INDICATIONS

The field of vertebroplasty and kyphoplasty is continuously evolving, and the authors recommend following the guidelines put forth by national and international societies.[20]

The main indications for vertebroplasty and kyphoplasty are (1) intractable, intense pain adjacent to the level of the fracture[9,10] in patients who have osteoporotic fractures diagnosed by radiographs, CT, or MRI. Conservative management for at least 3 to 4 weeks[21] should have failed in these patients for the surgical procedure to produce clinically relevant pain relief; and (2) pain of the affected segment in patients who have osteolytic changes of vertebral bodies from bony metastases.[20]

Contraindications to vertebroplasty and kyphoplasty are (1) unmanageable bleeding disorder, (2) improvement of symptoms with conservative management, (3) asymptomatic vertebral body fracture, (4) local or generalized infection, (5) allergy to bone cement, and (6) tumor mass with involvement of the spinal canal.

Vertebral augmentation as prophylaxis in patients who have osteoporosis is debated. It is regarded as a contraindication in some guidelines,[22] yet some investigators advocate vertebral augmentation for patients at very high risk for fracture.[23]

Retropulsion of a fragment into the spinal canal and a vertebral collapse of more than 70% of the height of the original vertebral body is no longer considered a contraindication. However, only experienced clinicians should perform a vertebroplasty on these patients.

The Consensus Guidelines for Vertebroplasty developed by the Standards of Practice Committee of the Society of Interventional Radiology[24,25] are (1) painful primary and secondary osteoporotic vertebral compression fractures refractory to medical therapy, (2) painful vertebrae with extensive osteolysis or invasion secondary to benign or malignant tumor, and (3) painful vertebral fracture associated with osteonecrosis.

TECHNIQUES
Vertebroplasty

To achieve a low complication rate, the most important factor influencing the outcome of the vertebroplasty is the visualization of needle placement and cement application.[26] Vertebroplasty may be performed using single-plane fluoroscopy, but the authors prefer to use CT scanning, which decreases the procedure time[27] and facilitates accurate visualization of needle placement and distribution of the cement. Monitoring cement distribution under direct fluoroscopic control is another crucial aspect of the procedure, independent of the technique used for needle placement (Figs. 1–5).

Vertebroplasty can be performed under local anesthesia only or a combination of conscious sedation[28] in most patients, and is therefore particularly useful in patients with risk factors for general anesthesia. General anesthesia is required only in patients unable to cooperate due to pain or extreme agitation.[29]

The access path depends on the level of the vertebral segment to be injected. In the lumbar spine, a transpedicular route is preferred; in the thoracic vertebrae, an intercostovertebral access is recommended; and in the cervical vertebrae, an anterolateral approach is used. Osteoporotic fractures normally do not occur in the cervical spine.

To identify potential routes of venous cement extravasation, an angiographic evaluation of the vertebral venous system (venography) has been suggested before cement injection, but its utility

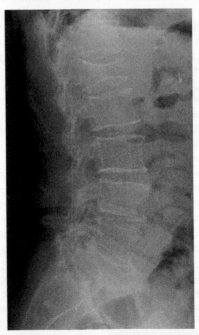

Fig. 1. Lateral radiograph in a 73-year-old male patient with back pain showing a vertebral fracture of the body of L1.

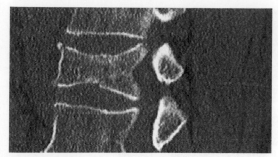

Fig. 2. Sagittal CT view showing the fracture of the first lumbar vertebra.

is still debated.[30–32] The cement should be injected while it is the consistency of toothpaste in order to minimize complications from extravasation in the surrounding tissues, as the flow characteristics of the cement change over time.

Cement injection may be stopped when the anterior two thirds of the vertebral body are filled and the cement is homogenously distributed between both endplates.[33] During cement injection, continuous fluoroscopic monitoring is performed to immediately detect extravasation of cement. In case of extravasation, the procedure must be immediately interrupted and the situation assessed. The vital parameters of the patient must be strictly monitored. In patients in whom extravasation of the cement determines neurological damages, open surgical decompression may be an option.

A direct correlation between the risk of extraosseous extravasation and the amount of cement injection has been proposed, but, to date, no studies have addressed the specific issue of the volume of cement needed during vertebroplasty. Normally, 2.5 to 4 mL of cement should provide adequate filling of the vertebra and achieve both consolidation and pain relief in patients who have

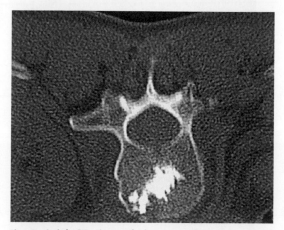

Fig. 3. Axial CT view of the vertebra after PMMA injection.

osteoporotic fractures. The materials cost of a single-level vertebroplasty is approximately 300 US dollars.[34]

Kyphoplasty

Kyphoplasty is normally performed under general anesthesia because proper placement of the inflatable bone tamp (ie, orthopedic balloon) is mandatory, and several steps need to be taken before cement can be injected.

A mono-, bilateral trans-, or parapedicular approach is used to insert a working cannula into the posterior aspect of the vertebral body. The procedure is performed under biplanar fluoroscopy or CT scan control. With reaming tools, two working channels within the anterior aspect of the vertebral body are produced, and the appropriate balloons are inserted. Ideally, the balloons should be centered between the two endplates in the anterior two thirds of the vertebral body. To obtain reduction of the fractured vertebra and to produce a cavity, the balloons are inflated using visual volume and pressure controls. The behavior of the vertebral body is monitored under fluoroscopic control. Inflation is stopped when a pressure above 250 psi is obtained, when the balloons contact the cortical surface of the vertebral body, or if the balloons expand beyond the border of the vertebral body, and if the height of the vertebra is restored. Successively, the balloons are retracted and PMMA is injected using a blunt cannula under continuous fluoroscopic control. The materials cost of a single-level kyphoplasty is approximately 4000 US dollars.[34]

PITFALLS

The procedures have a low rate of clinically relevant complications, but some can potentially be devastating, and should be discussed thoroughly with the patient and their family before the procedure. Cement extravasation is one of the possible complications of vertebroplasty. The reported incidence is up to 40% in patients who have osteoporotic fractures. Paravertebral soft tissue, intervertebral disc, needle tract, epidural and paravertebral veins, the spinal canal, and the neural foramen can be invaded. The clinical relevance of this complication depends on which anatomic structure is invaded by the cement. Cement invasion into the vena cava, lungs, heart, and even the kidneys have been described.[35–39] These major adverse events only occur in less than 1% of the patients,[40] and require immediate management.

In patients who have osteoporosis, new fractures of neighboring vertebrae can be caused by

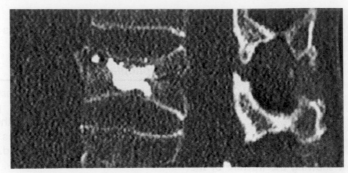

Fig. 4. Sagittal CT view of the vertebra after PMMA injection.

cement leakage within the intervertebral disc.[41] The pathogenesis of these new fractures is still under debate, and probably resides in the difference between the stiffness of the vertebra undergoing the procedure and the adjacent vertebral body.[38] Moreover, the high temperature of the cement during polymerization $(85°C)$[42] may cause thermal damage to the surrounding tissues.

Mechanical stabilization of the fractured vertebral body, chemical toxicity, and thermal necrosis of surrounding tissues and nerve endings have been indicated as the main reasons for pain relief after vertebroplasty.[13]

Vertebroplasty and kyphoplasty produce improvement in the quality of life for most patients because of pain relief, marked reduction of the amount of analgesics needed for pain control, and improvement in physical mobility.

As described above, an advantage of vertebroplasty over kyphoplasty is the ability to perform the procedure under local anesthesia only or a combination of conscious sedation[28] in most patients. For this reason, vertebroplasty is particularly useful in patients with risk factors for general anesthesia. General anesthesia is required only in patients unable to cooperate due to pain or extreme agitation.[29]

The rate of success in restoration of vertebral body height after kyphoplasty ranges from 0% to 90%. The incidence of leakage during kyphoplasty is reported to range from 0% to 13.5%,[11,43] and in vertebroplasty from 2% to 67%.[44–46] In addition to providing rapid pain relief, balloon kyphoplasty has the advantage of reducing acute fractures, allowing controlled cement placement under lower pressure, and improving deformity. Obviously, an elderly patient who has a vertebral compression fracture benefits greatly from restoration of normal overall spinal sagittal alignment and repair of kyphotic deformity.

Several authors have reported its effectiveness in pain relief and in preservation of posture.[47,48] Despite the high rate of successful outcomes

from vertebroplasty, this procedure does not restore the height of the vertebral body and does not correct kyphosis. Moreover, a low-viscosity cement injection technique is used, with a higher reported incidence of cement leakage when compared with kyphoplasty.[18,46,49,50]

VERTEBROPLASTY VERSUS KYPHOPLASTY: WHAT DOES THE AVAILABLE EVIDENCE SUGGEST?

Despite the good clinical outcomes reported with both vertebroplasty and kyphoplasty, and the fact that percutaneous vertebroplasty has been performed for more than 30 years, there is a lack of well-conducted randomized control trials on the subject. The evidence to support these techniques in the management of patients who have

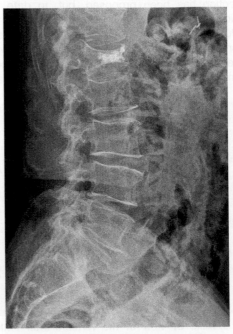

Fig. 5. Post-vertebroplasty lateral radiograph.

symptomatic osteoporotic vertebral compression fractures refractory to conventional medical therapy is, at best, based at Level III.[51,52] Three systematic reviews evaluated the efficacy and safety of vertebroplasty and kyphoplasty for the management of vertebral compression fractures.

Hulme and colleagues[53] performed a systematic literature review to evaluate the safety and efficacy of vertebroplasty and kyphoplasty with respect to pain relief, restoration of mobility and vertebral body height, complication rate, and incidence of new adjacent vertebral fractures. Many subjects experienced some pain relief—87% with vertebroplasty and 92% with kyphoplasty. Vertebral height restoration was possible using kyphoplasty and, for a subset of patients with mobile fractures, using vertebroplasty. Cement leaks occurred for 41% and 9% of treated vertebrae for vertebroplasty and kyphoplasty, respectively. New fractures of adjacent vertebrae occurred for both procedures at rates that are higher than the general osteoporotic population but approximately equivalent to the general osteoporotic population that had a previous vertebral fracture.

Taylor and colleagues[51,52] conducted a comparative systematic review of efficacy and safety of balloon kyphoplasty and vertebroplasty for the management of patients who have vertebral compression fractures. They concluded that, to date, there is no good-quality direct comparison between balloon kyphoplasty and vertebroplasty. From indirect comparison of case series evidence, the techniques seemed to provide similar pain relief, although for balloon kyphoplasty there is better documentation of gains in patient functionality and quality of life. The rates of adverse events (eg, pulmonary embolism, neurologic complications, and perioperative mortality) are low with both procedures, although poorly reported across studies.[51,52]

Ploeg and colleagues[19] undertook a systematic review to assess the efficacy and safety of percutaneous vertebroplasty in osteoporotic vertebral compression fractures. They reported on a total of 1136 interventions performed on 793 patients. The short-term complication rate ranged between 0.4% and 75.6%. Leakage of cement outside the vertebral body was markedly common, ranging from 3.3% to 75.6%. Although the majority were asymptomatic, a few devastating clinical adverse effects were reported. Percutaneous vertebroplasty is widely accepted for osteoporotic vertebral fractures, but the authors identified only one controlled trial. They concluded that there are insufficient data available to reliably assess efficacy of percutaneous vertebroplasty.

COSTS

Kyphoplasty is 10 to 20 times more expensive than vertebroplasty performed with conscious sedation on an outpatient basis.[27,30,54] Additional costs of a kyphoplasty include the device itself, the cost of the anesthesia, duration of the procedure, and inpatient hospitalization.[55]

CAUSES FOR CONCERN

Minimally invasive percutaneous vertebral augmentation methods for cement application into the vertebral body are potentially useful tools for the management of symptomatic compression fractures without neurologic impairment. However, they are not indicated for every type of fracture. External immobilization (ie, bracing or casting) remains the most important nonoperative management for vertebral fracture, and most patients will heal in a brace with nonoperative management.

A critical evaluation of the patient and the systematic use of computed tomography with sagittal and coronal reconstructions are necessary to avoid pitfalls in the diagnosis and successive management of patients who have vertebral fracture. If a spinal injury is detected, a CT scan and plain radiographs of the region should be obtained.

The decision to perform a cementoplasty depends on many factors, including being unable to carry out nonoperative treatment. such as the case of a vertebral fracture in an older patient who has cardiorespiratory disease, for whom extended bedrest, bracing or casting is not feasible.

Specific concerns of kyphoplasty include the fact that the endplates are not rigid structures. When the balloon is inflated, fissuration of the endplate may occur, with consequent extravasation into the intervertebral space. Moreover, when the fracture presents posterior fissuration, cement may invade the cord space, with dramatic neurologic damages. Cementoplasty techniques require skillful use of the cement, as its use in a liquid phase may cause embolism.

Another cause for concern is the postoperative presence of cement whose mechanical properties are different from those of vertebral bone. Although a minor problem in the limb surgery, it is of great concern in spinal surgery with respect to the neighboring structures.

In our clinical practice, the authors limit the use of cementoplasty to patients who have symptomatic compression fractures without neurologic impairment in whom a classical conservative management with bracing is not possible.

Although there are some patients for whom the benefits from vertebroplasty or kyphoplasty outweigh the risks, it is important to remember that successful conservative management of vertebral fractures has been the standard of care for many years.[56]

REFERENCES

1. Cook DJ, Guyatt GH, Adachi JD, et al. Quality of life issues in women with vertebral fractures due to osteoporosis. Arthritis Rheum 1993;36(6):750–6.
2. Gold DT. The clinical impact of vertebral fractures: quality of life in women with osteoporosis. Bone 1996;18(Suppl 3):185S–9S.
3. Phillips FM. Minimally invasive treatments of osteoporotic vertebral compression fractures. Spine 2003;28(Suppl 15):S45–53.
4. Dickman CA, Fessler RG, MacMillan M, et al. Transpedicular screw-rod fixation of the lumbar spine: operative technique and outcome in 104 cases. J Neurosurg 1992;77(6):860–70.
5. Esses SI, Sachs BL, Dreyzin V. Complications associated with the technique of pedicle screw fixation. A selected survey of ABS members. Spine 1993; 18(15):2231–8 [discussion: 2238–39].
6. Galibert P, Deramond H, Rosat P, et al. [Preliminary note on the treatment of vertebral angioma by percutaneous acrylic vertebroplasty]. Neurochirurgie 1987;33(2):166–8 [in French].
7. Garfin SR, Yuan HA, Reiley MA. New technologies in spine: kyphoplasty and vertebroplasty for the treatment of painful osteoporotic compression fractures. Spine 2001;26(14):1511–5.
8. Diamond TH, Bryant C, Browne L, et al. Clinical outcomes after acute osteoporotic vertebral fractures: a 2-year non-randomised trial comparing percutaneous vertebroplasty with conservative therapy. Med J Aust 2006;184(3):113–7.
9. Hoffmann RT, Jakobs TF, Ertl-Wagner BB, et al. [Vertebroplasty in osteoporotic vertebral compression]. Radiologe 2003;43(9):729–34 [in German].
10. Hoffmann RT, Jakobs TF, Wallnofer A, et al. [Percutaneous vertebroplasty (pv): indications, contraindications, and technique]. Radiologe 2003;43(9):709–17 [in German].
11. Fourney DR, Schomer DF, Nader R, et al. Percutaneous vertebroplasty and kyphoplasty for painful vertebral body fractures in cancer patients. J Neurosurg 2003;98(Suppl 1):21–30.
12. Lieberman IH, Dudeney S, Reinhardt MK, et al. Initial outcome and efficacy of "kyphoplasty" in the treatment of painful osteoporotic vertebral compression fractures. Spine 2001;26(14):1631–8.
13. Lieberman IH, Togawa D, Kayanja MM. Vertebroplasty and kyphoplasty: filler materials. Spine J 2005;5(Suppl 6):305S–16S.
14. Coumans JV, Reinhardt MK, Lieberman IH. Kyphoplasty for vertebral compression fractures: 1-year clinical outcomes from a prospective study. J Neurosurg 2003;99(Suppl 1):44–50.
15. Ledlie JT, Renfro M. Balloon kyphoplasty: one-year outcomes in vertebral body height restoration, chronic pain, and activity levels. J Neurosurg 2003;98(Suppl 1):36–42.
16. Siemionow K, Lieberman IH. Vertebral augmentation in osteoporosis and bone metastasis. Curr Opin Support Palliat Care 2007;1(4):323–7.
17. Phillips FM, Ho E, Campbell-Hupp M, et al. Early radiographic and clinical results of balloon kyphoplasty for the treatment of osteoporotic vertebral compression fractures. Spine 2003;28(19):2260–5 [discussion: 2265–67].
18. Phillips FM, Todd Wetzel F, Lieberman I, et al. An in vivo comparison of the potential for extravertebral cement leak after vertebroplasty and kyphoplasty. Spine 2002;27(19):2173–8 [discussion: 2178–79].
19. Ploeg WT, Veldhuizen AG, The B, et al. Percutaneous vertebroplasty as a treatment for osteoporotic vertebral compression fractures: a systematic review. Eur Spine J 2006;15(12):1749–58.
20. Gangi A, Sabharwal T, Irani FG, et al. Quality assurance guidelines for percutaneous vertebroplasty. Cardiovasc Intervent Radiol 2006;29(2):173–8.
21. Hide IG, Gangi A. Percutaneous vertebroplasty: history, technique and current perspectives. Clin Radiol 2004;59(6):461–7.
22. McGraw JK, Cardella J, Barr JD, et al. Society of Interventional Radiology quality improvement guidelines for percutaneous vertebroplasty. J Vasc Interv Radiol 2003;14(9 Pt 2):S311–5.
23. Kallmes DF, Jensen ME. Percutaneous vertebroplasty. Radiology 2003;229(1):27–36.
24. Fink A, Kosecoff J, Chassin M, et al. Consensus methods: characteristics and guidelines for use. Am J Public Health 1984;74(9):979–83.
25. McGraw JK, Cardella J, Barr JD, et al. Society of Interventional Radiology quality improvement guidelines for percutaneous vertebroplasty. J Vasc Interv Radiol 2003;14(7):827–31.
26. Laredo JD, Hamze B. Complications of percutaneous vertebroplasty and their prevention. Skeletal Radiol 2004;33(9):493–505.
27. Mathis JM. Percutaneous vertebroplasty. JBR-BTR 2003;86(5):299–301.
28. Gangi A, Guth S, Imbert JP, et al. Percutaneous vertebroplasty: indications, technique, and results. Radiographics 2003;23(2):e10.
29. White SM. Anaesthesia for percutaneous vertebroplasty. Anaesthesia 2002;57(12):1229–30.
30. Mathis JM. Percutaneous vertebroplasty: complication avoidance and technique optimization. AJNR Am J Neuroradiol 2003;24(8):1697–706.

31. Vasconcelos C, Gailloud P, Beauchamp NJ, et al. Is percutaneous vertebroplasty without pretreatment venography safe? Evaluation of 205 consecutive procedures. AJNR Am J Neuroradiol 2002;23(6): 913–7.

32. Deramond H, Depriester C, Galibert P, et al. Percutaneous vertebroplasty with polymethylmethacrylate. Technique, indications, and results. Radiol Clin North Am 1998;36(3):533–46.

33. Chavali R, Resijek R, Knight SK, et al. Extending polymerization time of polymethylmethacrylate cement in percutaneous vertebroplasty with ice bath cooling. AJNR Am J Neuroradiol 2003;24(3):545–6.

34. Armsen N, Boszczyk B. Vertebro-/kyphoplasty history, development, results. Eur J of Trauma 2005;31(5):433–41.

35. Quesada N, Mutlu GM. Images in cardiovascular medicine. Pulmonary embolization of acrylic cement during vertebroplasty. Circulation 2006;113(8): e295–6.

36. Barragan-Campos HM, Vallee JN, Lo D, et al. Percutaneous vertebroplasty for spinal metastases: complications. Radiology 2006;238(1):354–62.

37. Chung SE, Lee SH, Kim TH, et al. Renal cement embolism during percutaneous vertebroplasty. Eur Spine J 2006;15(Suppl 5):590–4.

38. Kim SH, Kang HS, Choi JA, et al. Risk factors of new compression fractures in adjacent vertebrae after percutaneous vertebroplasty. Acta Radiol 2004; 45(4):440–5.

39. Kim SY, Seo JB, Do KH, et al. Cardiac perforation caused by acrylic cement: a rare complication of percutaneous vertebroplasty. AJR Am J Roentgenol 2005;185(5):1245–7.

40. Nussbaum DA, Gailloud P, Murphy K. A review of complications associated with vertebroplasty and kyphoplasty as reported to the Food and Drug Administration medical device related web site. J Vasc Interv Radiol 2004;15(11):1185–92.

41. Uppin AA, Hirsch JA, Centenera LV, et al. Occurrence of new vertebral body fracture after percutaneous vertebroplasty in patients with osteoporosis. Radiology 2003;226(1):119–24.

42. Leeson MC, Lippitt SB. Thermal aspects of the use of polymethylmethacrylate in large metaphyseal defects in bone. A clinical review and laboratory study. Clin Orthop Relat Res 1993;(295):239–45.

43. Weisskopf M, Herlein S, Birnbaum K, et al. [Kyphoplasty - a new minimally invasive treatment for repositioning and stabilising vertebral bodies].

Z Orthop Ihre Grenzgeb 2003;141(4):406–11 [in German].

44. Cortet B, Cotten A, Boutry N, et al. Percutaneous vertebroplasty in the treatment of osteoporotic vertebral compression fractures: an open prospective study. J Rheumatol 1999;26(10):2222–8.

45. Ortiz AO, Zoarski GH, Beckerman M. Kyphoplasty. Tech Vasc Interv Radiol 2002;5(4):239–49.

46. Zoarski GH, Snow P, Olan WJ, et al. Percutaneous vertebroplasty for osteoporotic compression fractures: quantitative prospective evaluation of long-term outcomes. J Vasc Interv Radiol 2002;13(2 Pt 1):139–48.

47. Heini PF, Walchli B, Berlemann U. Percutaneous transpedicular vertebroplasty with PMMA: operative technique and early results. A prospective study for the treatment of osteoporotic compression fractures. Eur Spine J 2000;9(5):445–50.

48. Hodler J, Peck D, Gilula LA. Midterm outcome after vertebroplasty: predictive value of technical and patient-related factors. Radiology 2003;227(3): 662–8.

49. Mousavi P, Roth S, Finkelstein J, et al. Volumetric quantification of cement leakage following percutaneous vertebroplasty in metastatic and osteoporotic vertebrae. J Neurosurg 2003;99(Suppl 1):56–9.

50. Theodorou DJ, Theodorou SJ, Duncan TD, et al. Percutaneous balloon kyphoplasty for the correction of spinal deformity in painful vertebral body compression fractures. Clin Imaging 2002;26(1):1–5.

51. Taylor RS, Fritzell P, Taylor RJ. Balloon kyphoplasty in the management of vertebral compression fractures: an updated systematic review and meta-analysis. Eur Spine J 2007;16(8):1085–100.

52. Taylor RS, Taylor RJ, Fritzell P. Balloon kyphoplasty and vertebroplasty for vertebral compression fractures: a comparative systematic review of efficacy and safety. Spine 2006;31(23):2747–55.

53. Hulme PA, Krebs J, Ferguson SJ, et al. Vertebroplasty and kyphoplasty: a systematic review of 60 clinical studies. Spine 2006;31(17):1983–2001.

54. Mathis JM, Wong W. Percutaneous vertebroplasty: technical considerations. J Vasc Interv Radiol 2003;14(8):953–60.

55. Fergus E, McKiernan F. Kyphoplasty and vertebroplasty: how good is the evidence? Curr Rheumatol Rep 2007;1(9):57–65.

56. Longo UG, Denaro V. Spinal augmentation: what have we learnt? Lancet 2009;6;373(9679):1947;1947–8 [author reply].

The Anterolateral Minimally Invasive Approach for Total Hip Arthroplasty: Technique, Pitfalls, and Way Out

Erhan Basad, MD, PhD[a,*], Bernd Ishaque, MD, PhD[a],
Henning Stürz, MD, PhD[a], Jörg Jerosch, MD, MD (Hon), PhD[b]

KEYWORDS
- Minimally invasive • THA
- Anterolateral minimally invasive hip approach
- Total hip arthroplasty • ALMI

Minimally invasive surgery has reached the limelight and is praised for small skin incisions. In hip surgery, however, other structures are important for the functional outcome, and the length of the skin incision is not the only issue that attracts proponents of minimally invasive hip surgery. Although total hip arthroplasty (THA) is a successful procedure, some problems associated with it cause discomfort and negative results. These problems are mostly related to surgical trauma and include greater trochanter pain, early fatigue, and limping that can last up to 1 year after surgery. MRI after THA shows partial disruptions of the gluteus medius, with mucoid signal alterations and fatty degeneration even in asymptomatic patients.[1] Muscle protection seems to be the most important motivation for minimally invasive surgery of the hip. Shortcomings of classic THA techniques can be fixation strength, instability through muscle weakness, demineralization of bone through muscle detachment, and bone loss through resection. To improve THA techniques, surgeons have to question whether a minimally invasive surgical approach can address all these problems. Possible drawbacks of minimally

invasive approaches can be a less favorable field of vision, the necessity of introducing a new procedure that has several different surgical steps, higher rates in implant malpositioning, and soft tissue lesions through blunt trauma caused by the instruments.

Historically, the curved shape of the Müller banana stem and similar other stems allowed a muscle-preserving insertion over the anterolateral approach. Watson-Jones developed the anterolateral approach in 1936, which uses an interval between the tensor fascia latae muscle and the gluteus medius and minimus muscles. New cementless straight stems demanded a lateral transgluteal approach to allow reaming and insertion of the stem. In our clinic, the transgluteal lateral approach was the standard procedure for cemented and cementless stems. The transgluteal approach was first described by Bauer and Hardinge[2,3] in the late 1970s and early 1980s: the glutei muscles together with the vastus lateralis muscle are split along the fibers. The anterior parts of the muscle insertions are detached from the greater trochanter. This lateral approach

[a] Clinic & Polyclinic for Orthopaedic Surgery, University Hospital Giessen-Marburg GmbH, Paul-Meimberg-Strasse 3, 35392 Giessen, Germany
[b] Clinic for Orthopedics, Johanna-Etienne-Hospital, Am Hasenberg 46, 41462 Neuss, Germany
* Corresponding author.
E-mail address: erhan.basad@ortho.med.uni-giessen.de (E. Basad).

Orthop Clin N Am 40 (2009) 473–478
doi:10.1016/j.ocl.2009.05.001
0030-5898/09/$ – see front matter © 2009 Elsevier Inc. All rights reserved.

orthopedic.theclinics.com

is associated with two iatrogenic problems: limping attributable to abductor insufficiency and pain at the greater trochanter. These problems can result from injury to the inferior branch of the superior gluteus nerve and failure of the abductor repair.[4]

Our decision to use a minimally invasive approach in THA was influenced by the demand for minimal invasion in our surgical setup without prolongation of the learning curve and lesser muscle trauma. Different approaches, such as the two-incision lateral technique and the dorsolateral technique, have been described. After some time, it became obvious that the anterolateral approach was suitable because we could switch without essentially changing positioning of the patient and interfering with our familiar visualization of the surgical field.

Jerosch and colleagues[5] described this approach as the anterolateral minimally invasive (ALMI), which can be considered a reduced Watson-Jones approach. Jerosch and colleagues used the supine position on a standard table with a straight skin incision 6 to 8 cm anterior to the greater trochanter and described a different centering of the incision depending on varus or valgus deformities. Another minimally invasive version of the Watson-Jones approach was described by Bertin and Rottinger,[6] which is performed with the patient in a lateral position, with the incision directed from the greater trochanter toward the anterior superior iliac spine. The lateral decubitus position was preferred for the femoral preparation, which preferably can be performed in hyperextension-adduction and external rotation of the hip. Our preferred positioning is a supine position with a standard table. The following section describes the techniques and pitfalls that we encountered in our clinic and the ways in which we solved problems.

PATIENT POSITIONING AND DRAPING

Patients are placed in the supine position, with the axis of the pelvis lying at a right angle to the long axis of the table (**Fig. 1**). Orientation of the supine position and correction of leg length discrepancy during surgery are easily accomplished with this positioning. The greater trochanter has to lie 10 cm distal to the leg hinge on the table; it makes lowering of the contralateral leg during the figure-four position easier. The hip and lower limb are prepared and draped so that they can be moved freely during the procedure. Excellent muscle relaxation should be achieved using general or regional anesthesia.

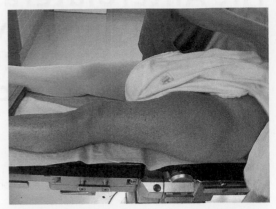

Fig. 1. Supine positioning on standard table with hinge 5 to 10 cm distally from greater trochanter.

SURGICAL EXPOSURE

The skin landmarks that must be identified are the greater trochanter and the anterior superior iliac spine. The skin incision is made slightly oblique, overlapping 2 to 3 cm distal to the greater trochanter and directing 30% upward to the anterior superior iliac spine, with a length of 6 to 10 cm, matching with the proximal one third of the Watson-Jones incision (**Fig. 2**). An oblique incision allows ease of pulling away soft tissue for visualizing the acetabulum. The fascia is exposed with skin retractors and opened longitudinally to the skin incision (**Fig. 3**). The iliotibial tract muscle is identified and retracted. If hypertrophic, the trochanteric bursa is excised as a possible source of postoperative pain. A fat tissue line between the gluteus muscle and the tensor muscle of fascia lata identifies the interval, which has to be opened by blunt dissection to approach the joint capsule (**Fig. 4**). A blunt Hohmann retractor is cautiously

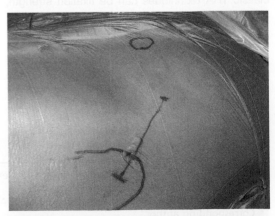

Fig. 2. Drawn landmarks, greater trochanter and anterior superior iliac spine. Oblique incision 6 to 10 cm, slightly overlapping the greater trochanter distally.

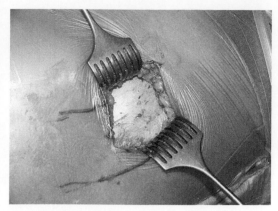

Fig. 3. Exposing of the fascia lata, which has to be opened longitudinally to the skin incision.

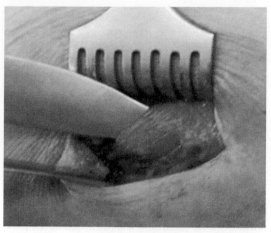

Fig. 5. Blunt dissection of interval and insertion of blunt Hohmann retractors.

placed under the gluteus medius, superior to the joint capsule, and blunt dissection is performed in this plane to the acetabular rim with a periosteal elevator. The second Hohmann retractor is placed ventromedially around the femoral neck, and the third one is placed at the anterior aspect of the acetabulum (**Fig. 5**). The capsule is incised in a reverse T shape and excised using diathermy to provide homeostasis. At this point, either the femoral head can be dislocated by adduction and external rotation or the neck can be osteotomized in situ (**Fig. 6**). The head can be dislocated out of the wound and prepared according to the implant to use. A resurfacing procedure is possible in this position, although additional axial pressure is necessary to keep the femoral head out of the wound.

ACETABULAR EXPOSURE AND PREPARATION

In case of a neck osteotomy, the femoral head is extracted and the limb with the femoral neck can

be retracted by placing a Hohmann retractor behind the posterior acetabulum, which is held by the first assistant who simultaneously applies traction on the limb. A second Hohmann retractor is placed at the anterior acetabulum and is held by the second assistant. The remaining capsule and limbus can be excised to allow acetabulum preparation for cup implantation in a standard fashion (**Fig. 7**). The incision window can be moved during cup preparation, which allows good three-dimensional orientation. With the minimally invasive approach, spherical cups are easier to insert than cone-shaped, sharp-threaded cups.

FEMORAL EXPOSURE AND PREPARATION

Hyperextension of the hip provides additionally better access to the proximal femur and is provided by lowering both legs of the table. The skin window has to be moved and the greater

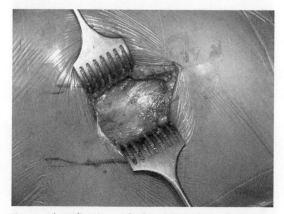

Fig. 4. Identification of the interval: a fatty line between tensor fascia lata and gluteus medius muscle.

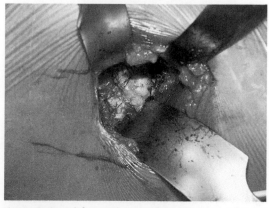

Fig. 6. Exposed femoral neck after resection of anterior capsule.

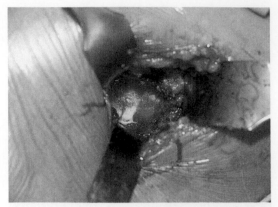

Fig. 7. Visualization of the acetabulum with three retractors after osteotomy and retraction of the proximal femur.

trochanter is delivered into the approach using a Hohmann retractor, which displaces the iliotibial tract dorsally. A second blunt Hohmann retractor is placed anteriorly in the area of the lesser trochanter. The second assistant holds the limb in adduction and external rotation. At this point, the capsular attachments at the dorsolateral part of the proximal femur are tensioned, and this tension can be perceived in the proximal femur. Careful dissection with the diathermy stick should be performed with simultaneous adduction and external rotation. If the proximal femur is exposed, the femoral canal can be prepared in the usual fashion (**Fig. 8**). It is important that the gluteus medius and the external rotators be preserved.

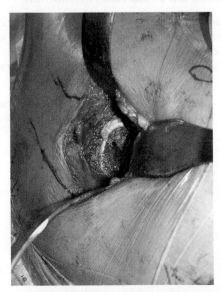

Fig. 8. Visualization of proximal femur after release of the dorsal capsule in adduction and external rotation. Both legs are lowered to provide hyperextension.

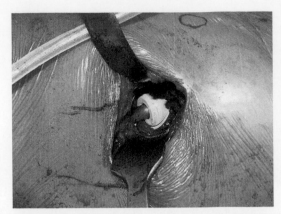

Fig. 9. Surgical field after implantation and reduction of the prosthetic joint.

Excessive prolonged pressure on the soft tissues by the retractors increases the risk of nerve injuries and muscle degeneration dramatically. Trial reduction with adjusting of the leg length can be accomplished easily in the supine position (**Fig. 9**).

WOUND CLOSURE

Because there is no muscle transection, simple juxtaposition of the interval between vastus lateralis and gluteus medius and closure of the iliotibial muscle is performed (**Fig. 10**). Subcutaneous tissue and skin are closed in layers. A single intra-articular suction drain is sufficient in ordinary cases (**Fig. 11**). If a thick subcutaneous layer is present, a second drain helps to prevent a subcutaneous hematoma.

DEDICATED INSTRUMENTS

Although not absolutely necessary, several specially adapted minimally invasive surgery

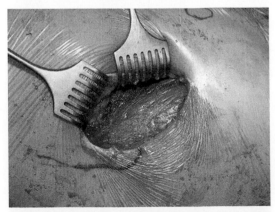

Fig. 10. Muscle interval adapts spontaneously after removing retractors. The gluteus medius muscle remains without macroscopic damage.

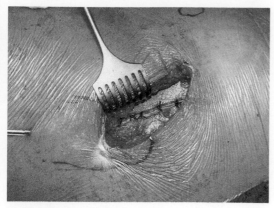

Fig. 11. Closure of fascia lata after insertion of a single joint suction drain.

instruments are helpful in this approach. An angled cup reamer and angled Hohmann retractors help to prepare the acetabulum. A trochanter retractor with two prongs also helps to elevate the proximal femur into the wound (**Fig. 12**).

PITFALLS AND SOLUTIONS

We have encountered several pitfalls, one of which is hemorrhage from posterior retracted capsule out of sight of the surgeon. The surgeon can avoid uncontrolled bleeding in a narrow environment by using a long-handled diathermy stick during capsule resection. If bleeding occurs, typically during soft tissue release before femur preparation, the surgeon should pull the femur laterally and rotate externally to expose the dorsal capsule. Another pitfall involves trochanter avulsion during approach of the figure-four position. At this critical point of the surgery, an insufficient release of dorsal capsule attachments and ineffective muscle relaxation can cause this complication.

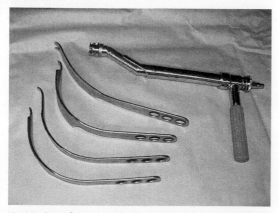

Fig. 12. Set of recommended instruments: angled cup reamer, angled Hohman retractors (30°, 45°, and 90°).

The surgeon must be sure to release the soft tissues appropriately when exposing the proximal femur. If the iliotibial tract cannot be displaced sufficiently despite good muscle relaxation, a horizontal incision into the iliotibial tract may help to increase the adduction of the limb.

DISCUSSION

There still is no generally accepted common definition for minimally invasive hip surgery, but mainly it is correct to say that decreased soft tissue trauma is the main goal. The anterior approaches are commonly used, provide lower dislocation rates, and allow good acetabular exposure. On the other hand, anterior approaches temporarily show a higher rate of limping from abductor weakening and slightly higher blood loss, compared with lateral approaches.[7,8] Hip dislocation is a major complication after total hip surgery.[9] In hip approaches, the main cause of dislocation is insufficiency of the abductor muscles. Muscles also play a major role in bone preservation. Hasart and colleagues[10] performed bone densitometries after THA and evaluated the proximal femur according to the Green classification. They showed that muscle trauma during THA indicates significant bone demineralization.

The anterolateral approach has been modified to decrease gluteus medius disruption and results in the currently used anterolateral minimally invasive surgical techniques. Current studies comparing open and mini-incision techniques have found statistically significant advantages in blood loss, limping, and length of hospital stay.[5,11–14] In contrast, other authors saw no significant differences in open versus mini-open techniques[11–14] but imply that the learning curve may influence the outcome in newly adopted techniques, even for experienced surgeons.

Among the approaches in the supine position, the ALMI approach to the hip provides a muscle-preserving technique and is suitable for all developments in total hip replacement. Unlike in the posterior approach, resection of the anterior capsule in the ALMI technique does not increase the risk of hip dislocation. Tenotomies do not affect the sensimotor capabilities of the joint, and the anterolateral approach provides easy access for revision surgery. The ALMI surgical approach that we present is derived from the conventional Watson-Jones approach and is an extensile approach. It is safe and reproducible and does not require specialized instruments or implants, although we acknowledge that custom-made instrumentation may make the procedure easier. In our hands, the ALMI technique fulfills the main goals of minimal trauma by preserving the abductor muscle and dorsal capsule. The learning curve is an important issue, even for experienced surgeons. Switching from our standard, conventional, open lateral approach to the ALMI approach occurred in a smooth and safe transition without technique-related complications, simultaneously fulfilling the essential goals of minimally invasive THA.

REFERENCES

1. Pfirrmann CA, Notzli HP, Dora C, et al. Abductor tendons and muscles assessed at MR imaging after total hip arthroplasty in asymptomatic and symptomatic patients. Radiology 2005;235:969–76.
2. Hardinge K. The direct lateral approach to the hip. J Bone Joint Surg Br 1982;64:17–9.
3. Bauer R, Kerschbaumer F, Poisel S, Oberthaler W. The transgluteal approach to the hip joint. Arch Orthop Trauma Surg 1979;95(1,2):47–9.
4. Stähelin T. Abduktorennahtversagen und nervenschädigung beim transglutealen zugang zur hüfte. [Abductor repair failure and nerve damage during hip replacement via the transgluteal approach]. Orthopäde 2006;35:1215–24.
5. Jerosch J, Theising C, Fadel ME. Antero-lateral minimal invasive (ALMI) approach for total hip arthroplasty technique and early results. Arch Orthop Trauma Surg 2006;126:164–73.
6. Bertin KC, Rottinger H. Antero-lateral mini-incision hip replacement surgery: a modified Watson Jones approach. Clin Orthop Relat Res 2004;429:248–55.
7. Roberts JM, Fu FH, McClain EJ. A comparison of the posterolateral and anterolateral approaches to total hip arthroplasty. Clin Orthop 1984;187:205–10.
8. Vicar AJ, Coleman CR. A comparison of the antero-lateral, transtrochanteric, and posterior surgical approaches in primary total hip arthroplasty. Clin Orthop 1984;188:152–69.
9. Hedlundh U, Ahnfelt L, Hybbinette CH. Surgical experience related to dislocation after total hip arthroplasty. J Bone Joint Surg Br 1996;78:206–9.
10. Hasart O, Hanebeck J, Labs K, et al. Periprothetische knöcherne Veränderungen 2, 4 und 6 Jahre nach Implantation zementfrei verankerter Zweymüller-schäfte-eine Querschnittsstudie [Periprosthetic osseous changes 2, 4, and 6 years after implantation of cementless Zweymüller-stems - a cross-sectional study]. Z Orthop Ihre Grenzgeb 2002;140(3):323–7 [in German].
11. Goldstein WM, Branson JJ, Berland KA, et al. Minimal-incision total hip arthroplasty. J Bone Joint Surg Am 2003;85(4):33–8.
12. Nakamura S, Matsuda K, Arai N, et al. Mini-incision posterior approach for total hip arthroplasty. Int Orthop 2004;28(4):214–7.
13. Chimento GF, Pavone V, Sharrock NE, et al. Minimal invasive total hip arthroplasty: a prospective randomized study. Paper presented at the 70th Annual meeting of the American Academy of Orthopedic Surgeons. New Orleans, August 2, 2003.
14. Mahmood A, Zafar MS, Majid I, et al. Minimally invasive hip arthroplasty: a quantitative review of the literature. Br Med Bull 2007;84:37–48.

Minimally Invasive Total Knee Arthroplasty: A Systematic Review

Anil Khanna, MRCS, MS (Ortho)[a,b],
Nikolaos Gougoulias, MD, PhD, CCST (Ortho)[a],
Umile Giuseppe Longo, MD[c],
Nicola Maffulli, MD, MS, PhD, FRCS (Orth)[d,*]

KEYWORDS
- Arthroplasty • Knee • Minimally invasive surgery
- Total joint replacement

The history of total joint replacement has demonstrated continuous evolution. The relatively high complication rates associated with early prostheses models and techniques eventually led to the improvement of implants and refinement of the surgical procedures. Gradual adoption of these improvements and their diffusion led to increased success rates of implantation.[1]

With the development of total knee arthroplasty (TKA) since 1974, this field has undergone many changes.[2,3] Despite outstanding results,[4,5] many patients experience pain and impaired quadriceps muscle function in the short-term with prolonged rehabilitative efforts until full recovery.[6] Mizner and colleagues[7] analyzed 40 subjects who underwent unilateral TKA followed by rehabilitation, including 6 weeks of outpatient physical therapy. In their study, subjects experienced significant worsening of range of motion, quadriceps strength, and performance on functional tests 1 month after surgery. Of all physical measures assessed, quadriceps muscle strength showed the greatest decline, and was the most highly correlated measure associated with functional performance at all testing sessions. Likewise, Silva and colleagues[8] assessed quadriceps muscle strength by measuring isometric extension peak torque in 32 knees more than 2 years after TKA. The mean isometric extension peak torque values in their subjects were reduced by up to 30.7% ($P = .01$), and the isometric flexion peak torque values were 32.2% lower than those from control subjects.

With the evolution of minimally invasive surgery for unicondylar knee arthroplasty in early 1990s and in an effort to reduce quadriceps muscle strength loss with improved clinical outcome (eg, reduced pain, reduced length of hospitalization, and earlier return to full function) following TKA, minimally invasive quadriceps-sparing techniques were introduced.[9-14]

Proponents of such techniques suggested faster recovery times, less pain and improved cosmesis for their patients,[15,16] whereas critics cite reduced visualization as a risk for poorer component placement that could compromise long-term survivorship of the prosthesis.[17]

We performed a systematic review of the published literature on Minimally Invasive Total Knee Arthroplasty (MITKA), and analyzed the reported surgical outcomes.

[a] Department of Trauma and Orthopaedic Surgery, Keele University School of Medicine, University Hospital of North Staffordshire, Stoke-on-Trent, Staffordshire ST4 7QB, UK
[b] DePuy International Implant Research Fellow, University Hospital of North Staffordshire, Hartshill Road, Stoke-on-Trent, Staffordshire ST4 7PA, UK
[c] Department of Orthopaedic and Trauma Surgery, Campus Biomedico University, Via Alvaro del Portillo, 200, Rome 00128, Italy
[d] Centre for Sports and Exercise Medicine, Barts and The London School of Medicine and Dentistry, Queen Mary University of London, Mile End Hospital, 275 Bancroft Road, London E1 4DG, UK
* Corresponding author.
E-mail address: n.maffulli@qmul.ac.uk (N. Maffulli).

Orthop Clin N Am 40 (2009) 479–489
doi:10.1016/j.ocl.2009.05.003
0030-5898/09/$ – see front matter © 2009 Elsevier Inc. All rights reserved.

orthopedic.theclinics.com

MATERIALS AND METHODS
Literature Search and Data Extraction

We performed a comprehensive search of PubMed, Medline, Cochrane, CINAHL, and Embase databases using various combinations of the keywords: minimally invasive total knee arthroplasty, mini-incision total knee replacement and minimally invasive arthroplasty. All articles relevant to the subject were retrieved and their bibliographies searched for further references in context to MITKA. The search was limited to articles published in peer-reviewed journals in English.

We excluded case reports, literature reviews, letter to editors and articles not specifically reporting outcomes. Studies using navigation-assisted MITKA were excluded from the review, as it is a different, separate surgical technique.

From each article, two investigators (AK and NG) independently extracted the year of publication, type of study (ie, randomized controlled trial, prospective study, or retrospective case series), number of implanted joints, length of follow-up, incision length, blood loss, tourniquet time, postoperative pain, length of hospital stay, range of motion, supplementary unplanned procedures, complications (ie, component malalignment, wound healing problems, superficial and deep infections), and prosthesis survival (with revision as an endpoint).

Methodological Quality Assessment

The Coleman methodology score (CMS),[18,19] which was originally developed for and used to grade clinical studies on cartilage repair and patellar or Achilles tendinopathy, and subsequently used in several other systematic reviews,[20–22] was adapted to evaluate studies reporting on MITKA (**Table 1**). This scoring system assesses methodology using the 10 criteria, giving a total score between 0 and 100. A score approaching 100 indicates that the study has a robust design and largely avoids chance, various biases, or confounding factors. A score greater than 85 is considered excellent; 70 to 84, good; 50 to 69, moderate; and less than 50, poor.[18] The subsections that compose the CMS are based on the subsections of the CONSORT statement (for randomized controlled trials),[23] but are modified to allow for other trial designs. Two investigators (AK and NG) independently scored the quality of the studies. Each investigator scored the quality of the studies twice, with a time interval of 3 weeks between each scoring session to minimize intraobserver error. Intra- and interobserver reliability was examined. Where differences were encountered, agreement was achieved by consensus.

The presented scores are those that were set by agreement of both examiners.

Statistical Methods

To assess reliability of quality scoring using the CMS, intraclass correlations for interobserver[24] and the Spearman–Brown coefficient[25] for intraobserver reliability were used. Student's t-test was used compare means of CMS between the two examiners. Student's t-test was also used to compare means of CMS for different implants. Odds ratio and confidence intervals (95%) were calculated where pooling of data was appropriate. The level of statistical significance was 0.05. We used SPSS version 14.0 for Windows (SPSS Inc., Chicago, Illinois) for statistical analyses.

RESULTS
Studies

Initial databases search retrieved 85 studies; of these, 46 studies were excluded because they did not report on outcome of MITKA. Eight studies were in a language other than English. Of the three studies (Tanavalee and colleagues,[26] Schroer and colleagues,[27] and Berger and colleagues[28]) with overlapping publication of data, only the latest publication was considered. This left 28 studies, published from January 2003 to June 2008, to be included in the present investigation. Of these 28 studies, there were four prospective randomized control trials, 14 prospective studies (including one randomized on two different approaches for MITKA) and 10 retrospective studies. Of the 28 studies, 18 were comparison studies between standard approach and minimally invasive approach, and 10 studies reported on outcomes of MITKA alone.

Demographics Details

Twenty-eight studies included in the study reported on 2648 MITKA and 848 standard approach total knee arthroplasty (STKA). The age range of subjects in the MITKA group ranged from 63 to 76 years, whereas the age range in STKA group ranged from 63 to 73.9 years. In the MITKA group, there were 1605 women and 1043 men, and in the STKA group there were 560 women and 288 men. Osteoarthritis was the primary diagnosis in both groups (2524 of 2648 subjects in the MITKA group, and 781 of 848 in the STKA group). Inflammatory arthropathies formed the rest of the subject population in both groups, though four studies excluded subjects who had inflammatory arthropathies.[29–32] The follow-up of subjects ranged from 1.5 months to 36 months postoperatively.

Table 1
Modified Coleman methodology score

Part A: Only One Score to be Given for Each of the 7 Sections		
1. Study size — number of MITKA	< 30	0
	30–50	4
	51–100	7
	> 100	10
2. Mean follow-up	< 12 mo	0
	12–36 mo	4
	37–60 mo	7
	> 61 mo	10
3. Surgical approach	Different approach used and outcome not reported separately	0
	Different approaches used and outcome reported separately	7
	Single approach used	10
4. Type of study	Retrospective cohort study	0
	Prospective cohort study	10
	Randomized control trial	15
5. Description of indications/diagnosis (OA, RA, etc.)	Described without % specified	0
	Described with % specified	5
6. Descriptions of surgical technique	Inadequate (not stated, unclear)	0
	Fair (technique only stated)	5
	Adequate (technique stated, details of surgical procedure given)	10
7. Description of postoperative rehabilitation	Described	5
	Not described	0
Part B: Scores May be Given for Each Option in Each of the 3 Sections if Applicable		
1. Outcome criteria	Outcome measures clearly defined	2
	Timing of outcome assessment clearly stated	2
	Use of outcome criteria that has reported reliability	3
	General health measure included	3
2. Procedure of assessing outcomes	Subjects recruited	5
	Investigator independent of surgeon	4
	Written assessment	3
	Completion of assessment by subjects themselves with minimal investigator assistance	3
3. Description of subject selection process	Selection criteria reported and unbiased	5
	Recruitment rate reported	
	> 90%	5
	= 90%	0

Quality Assessment

The mean CMS calculated for the 28 studies included in the present investigation was 60 (SD 9.26; 95% CI 55.8-62.7), characterized as moderate. There was no significant difference between the mean CMS of the two examiners (59.5 compared with 61.5, P = .83). Intraobserver Spearman–Brown coefficient was 0.90, and the intraclass correlation was 0.84, indicating substantial agreement. Disagreement occurred in eight studies (one parameter in each study). The values presented in (**Table 2**) are those set by agreement between the two examiners. Quality scores were good in 2, moderate in 25, and poor in 3 studies.

Incision length

Historically, MITKA was defined as an incision length of less than 14 cm.[14] Incision length was reported in 22 studies (2068 knees) in the MITKA

Table 2
Level of evidence and Coleman methodology scoring for the studies under review

No	Study (References)	Level of Evidence	Year of Publication	Procedures	Approach	No. of Knees (MITKA/STKA)	CMS
1	Han[40]	Prospective randomized	2008	MITKA v STKA	mini-parapatellar	30/30	69
2	Karachalios[29]	Prospective randomized	2008	MITKA v STKA	mini-midvastus	50/150	71
3	Chotanaphuti[41]	Prospective randomized	2008	MITKA v STKA	mini-parapatellar	20/20	65
4	Kashyap[48]	Prospective	2008	MITKA v STKA	mini-subvastus	25/25	68
5	Schroer[56]	Prospective	2008	MITKA v STKA	mini-subvastus	150/150	58
6	McAllister[30]	Prospective	2008	MITKA v STKA	mini-parapatellar	91/98	65
7	Tanavalee[26]	Prospective	2007	MITKA	mini-parapatellar	114	68
8	Tashiro[37]	Prospective	2007	MITKA v STKA	mini-parapatellar	24	56
9	Huang[33]	Prospective	2007	MITKA v STKA	mini-parapatellar	32/35	52
10	Sleyer[53]	Prospective	2007	MITKA	lateral approach	35	67
11	King[35]	Retrospective	2007	MITKA v STKA	mini-midvastus	100/50	41
12	Kolisek[34]	Prospective randomized	2007	MITKA v STKA	mini-midvastus	40/40	62
13	Schroer[27]	Retrospective	2007	MITKA v STKA	mini-subvastus	725/7	58
14	Chen[44]	Retrospective	2006	MITKA	mini-parapatellar	41/46	65
15	Shankar[42]	Prospective	2006	MITKA v STKA	mini-midvastus	102/76	64
16	Haas[50]	Retrospective	2006	MITKA	mini-midvastus	40/40	63
17	Aglietti[51]	Prospective randomized only for MITKA	2006	MITKA	Quadriceps-sparing v mini-subvastus	60	68
18	Pagnano[52]	Retrospective	2006	MITKA	subvastus approach	103	59
19	Berger[28]	Prospective	2006	MITKA	mini-parapatellar	100	50
20	Dalury[36]	Retrospective	2005	MITKA v STKA	midvastus	30/30	48
21	Tenholder[38]	Retrospective	2005	MITKA v STKA	mini-midvastus	69/49	58
22	Laskin[32]	Prospective	2005	MITKA	mini-midvastus	100	70
23	Boerger[31]	Prospective	2005	MITKA v STKA	mini-subvastus	60/60	67
24	Berger[43]	Prospective	2005	MITKA	mini-midvastus	50	60
25	Laskin[39]	Retrospective	2004	MITKA v STKA	mini-midvastus	32/26	43
26	Haas[55]	Prospective	2004	MITKA v STKA	mini-midvastus	40/40	55
27	Bonutti[54]	Retrospective	2003	MITKA	mini-midvastus	20	36
28	Tria[49]	Retrospective	2003	MITKA	mini-midvastus	70	53

group (range 7–14 cm). In the STKA group, the incision length was reported in all 18 studies (range 13.4–21 cm). This difference in the length of incision was reported as significant.[29–31,33–36]

Blood loss

Blood loss was reported in 11 studies (431 knees) in the MITKA group (range 108–1040 mL) and in 9 studies (235 knees) in the STKA group (range 110–1140 mL). Most of these studies (**Table 3**) report the loss of blood and decrease in postoperative hemoglobin in the MITKA group[29,37–40] as significantly less than the STKA group, the one exception being the study by Laskin and colleagues,[39] which reported higher blood loss in the MITKA group.

Tourniquet time

Most studies[29,33,34,38,40] on MITKA tend to report longer tourniquet time with this procedure compared with STKA, with the exception of the study by Chotanaphuti and colleagues,[41] who reported a mean operative duration of 50 minutes in the MITKA group as compared with 55 minutes in the STKA group. All authors report that as the experience of the operating surgeon with MITKA increases, the tourniquet time gradually decreases.[26,35,42]

Postoperative pain

Studies[30,31,33,35,37,39] reporting on postoperative pain and analgesic needs reported significant less pain with minimally invasive approach with lesser use of stronger analgesics 24 hours postoperatively as compared with STKA, with the exception of a prospective randomized controlled trial by Karachalios and colleagues,[29] who report higher pain in the MITKA group.

Duration of hospital stay

Most comparative studies reporting on hospital stay show shorter inpatient stay in MITKA group compared with STKA (see **Table 3**). Berger and colleagues[43] report discharging 99% of the subjects after 24 hours. The difference between the two groups was critically examined in only two studies,[43,44] and it was determined that it could result from a combination of early physiotherapy input and special anesthetic protocols[45–47] along with the minimally invasive approach.

Range of motion and quadriceps muscle strength restoration

The range of motion of the knee improved significantly in the postoperative period in both groups in comparison to preoperative values. Most studies comparing MITKA with conventional arthroplasty report better range of motion in the

MITKA group in the early postoperative period.[26,27,36,41,42] However, several studies following this variable closely over time report little or no difference between the two groups in subsequent follow-ups,[29–31,33,39,48] with the exception of study by Schroer and colleagues,[27] in which they report that the increased range of motion in the MITKA group is maintained over a 2-year follow-up period, although they did not record the STKA group range of motion beyond 1 year, making it difficult to state whether there really was a difference between the two groups. A consistent finding, however, is the quick recovery of quadriceps strength and earlier achievement of first 90° range of motion in the MITKA group.[28,40,49–54] Also, Han and colleagues[40] reported that MITKA may benefit patients undergoing simultaneous bilateral procedures with faster functional recovery in bilateral cases.

Knee scores

Most comparative studies reporting on the Knee Society Scoring either found no difference between the two groups, or the difference, if recorded, was limited to the initial postoperative period only.[29,30,32,33,37,39,44,55]

Complications

Component malalignment

Component malalignment (**Tables 4** and **5**) was documented in 58 of 571 knees in 10 studies of MITKA (range 0.8%–31%). In the STKA group, the malalignment of components was reported in 19 of 241 knees in 5 studies (range 0.4%–10.8%). Several studies report significantly high rates of malalignment in the MITKA group as a result of poor visualization of anatomic landmarks with the minimally invasive approach.[29,36,39,56]

Delayed wound healing

Wound-healing problems (see **Tables 4** and **5**) were reported in 12 studies with 1429 subjects in the MITKA group (range 0.5%–8.7%). In the STKA group, delayed wound healing was reported in 3 studies with 215 subjects (range 2.2%–5.3%). Delayed wound healing is higher in MITKA in several studies,[26,29,45,56] possibly from the excessive retraction during the procedure to improve visualization.

Superficial and deep infection

In the MITKA group, 7 studies involving 437 subjects reported superficial infection in 8 subjects (range 0.7%–8%), whereas in the STKA group, the rate of superficial infection was reported in 5 studies of 240 knees (range 1%–4%).

Table 3
Blood loss, tourniquet time, and duration of hospital stay in MITKA and STKA groups

Author	Year of Publication	Blood Loss (in ml)		Tourniquet Time (in Minutes)		Duration of Hospital Stay (in Days)	
		MITKA	STKA	MITKA	STKA	MITKA	STKA
McAllister	2008	—	—	65.7	71.1	3.6	6.4
Han	2008	609	871	77	63	—	—
Kashyap	2008	—	—	68	52	5.5	5.5
Chotanaphuti	2008	540	580	50	55	3.4	4.5
Karachalios	2008	613	1016	75	55	—	—
Schroer	2008	—	—	78	74	3.4	4.1
Huang	2007	—	—	122	55	—	—
Tanavalee	2007	470	—	110.3	—	3	—
Kolisek	2007	108	110	69	59	4	4.5
King	2007	—	—	86.3	78.9	2.8	3.7
Tashiro	2007	—	—	152	96	—	—
Seyler	2007	—	—	—	—	—	—
Schroer	2007	—	—	57	57	—	—
Shankar	2006	—	—	81	52	4.5	5.6
Haas	2006	—	—	55.5	—	—	—
Aglietti	2006	832	—	83	—	—	—
Chen	2006	246	249	108	51	3.1	5.9
Berger	2006	—	—	104	—	1	—
Pagnano	2006	—	—	58	—	2.8	—
Berger	2005	—	—	108	—	1	—
Tenholder	2005	292	638	81.7	82.9	3.9	4.2
Boerger	2005	1040	1140	81	64	—	—
Dalury	2005	—	—	31	32.4	—	—
Laskin	2005	—	—	56	—	—	—
Laskin	2004	713	573	58	51	—	—
Haas	2004	—	—	63	49	—	—
Bonutti	2003	—	—	—	—	2	—
Tria	2003	210	—	—	—	4	—

Table 4
Complications in MITKA group

Author	Year of Publication	Component Malalignment	Delayed Healing	Deep Infection	Superficial Infection	Revision	Manipulation Under Anesthesia	Conversion to Standard Approach
McAllister	2008	—	—	—	—	—	4	2
Berger	2006	—	—	—	1	—	2	—
Kashyap	2008	—	—	—	2	1	—	—
Karachalios	2008	6	4	—	—	—	1	6
Chotanaphuti	2008	—	—	—	1	—	—	—
Han	2008	—	2	—	—	—	—	—
Schroer	2008	—	7	2	1	2	1	—
Tanavalee	2007	1	10	—	—	—	—	—
Kolisek	2007	—	4	—	—	1	—	—
King	2007	16	—	—	—	—	1	—
Tashiro	2007	4	1	—	—	—	—	—
Seyler	2007	—	—	—	—	2	2	—
Schroer	2007	—	31	2	—	4	—	—
Huang	2007	9	2	—	—	—	—	—
Pagnano	2006	—	2	—	—	—	—	—
Shankar	2006	—	—	—	2	—	1	—
Haas	2006	—	2	2	—	2	8	—
Aglietti	2006	—	—	—	—	—	—	5
Chen	2006	13	—	—	—	—	—	—
Boerger	2005	1	—	—	—	—	—	—
Dalury	2005	4	3	—	—	—	—	—
Laskin	2005	3	—	—	—	—	—	—
Berger	2005	—	3	—	1	—	—	—
Tenholder	2005	—	—	—	—	—	—	—
Laskin	2004	—	—	—	—	—	—	—
Haas	2004	—	—	—	1	—	1	—
Tria	2003	—	—	—	—	—	—	2
Bonutti	2003	1	—	—	—	—	—	—

Table 5
Complications in the STKA group

Author	Year of Publication	Component malalignment	Delayed Healing	Deep Infection	Superficial Infection	Revision	Manipulation Under Anesthesia
McAllister	2008	—	—	—	1	—	16
Kashyap	2008	—	1	—	1	—	—
Chotanaphuti	2008	—	—	—	—	—	—
Karachalios	2008	2	—	—	1	—	—
Han	2008	—	—	—	—	—	—
Schroer	2008	—	6	2	—	2	—
Tanavalee	2007	—	—	—	—	—	—
Kolisek	2007	—	1	—	—	—	—
King	2007	7	—	—	—	—	—
Seyler	2007	—	—	—	—	—	—
Schroer	2007	—	—	—	—	—	—
Tashiro	2007	—	—	—	—	—	—
Huang	2007	2	—	—	—	—	—
Shankar	2006	—	—	—	2	—	1
Berger	2006	—	—	—	—	—	—
Haas	2006	—	—	—	—	—	—
Aglietti	2006	—	—	—	—	—	—
Pagnano	2006	—	—	—	—	—	—
Chen	2006	5	—	—	—	—	1
Boerger	2005	3	—	—	—	—	—
Dalury	2005	—	—	—	—	—	—
Laskin	2005	—	—	—	—	—	—
Berger	2005	—	—	—	—	—	—
Tenholder	2005	—	—	—	—	—	2
Laskin	2004	—	—	—	—	—	—
Haas	2004	—	—	—	1	—	3
Tria	2003	—	—	—	—	—	—
Bonutti	2003	—	—	—	—	—	—

In the MITKA group, deep infections in 6 subjects were reported in 3 studies involving 485 knees (range 0.2%–1.3%). In the STKA group, deep infections in 2 subjects were reported in 1 study of 150 knees (1.3%). These rates are not statistically different (see **Tables 4** and **5**).

Revision surgery
Implant failure leading to revision was reported in 12 subjects in 6 studies involving 1270 knees in the MITKA group (range 0.5%–5.7%). Causes of failure were deep infections in 6 subjects, component malalignment in 3, nerve injury in 1, and periprosthetic fracture in 2 subjects. In the STKA group, revision was reported in 2 subjects in 1 study with 190 knees (range 0.6%–2.5%). The

cause of both revisions was deep infection. The difference was not significant (see **Tables 4** and **5**).

Conversion of minimally invasive approach to standard approach
Four studies reported 11 conversions out of 271 subjects (range 2%–12%). Conversion from MITKA to STKA was performed when visualization became difficult, especially in obese subjects or subjects who had a severe deformity (see **Tables 4** and **5**).

Additional complications and additional procedures
Peroneal nerve palsy was reported in the MITKA group in 4 subjects in 3 studies of 174 knees

(range 1.1%–5.5%). In the STKA group, peroneal nerve palsy was seen in 1 subject in a series of 89 knees (1.1%).[30] There was one patellar tendon rupture in each group; MITKA group (1.6% in a group of 60 knees)[31] and STKA group (0.6% in a group of 150 knees).[56] There was one patellar fracture in a series of 725 cases in the MITKA group (0.01%).[56] Periprosthetic fractures were reported in 3 subjects in 3 studies[27,31,34] involving 250 knees in the MITKA group (range 0.6%–2%). In the STKA group, there was one periprosthetic fracture in a series of 150 subjects (0.06%).[27]

In the MITKA group, manipulation under anesthesia was reported in 21 subjects in 9 studies of 1003 subjects (range 0.6%–5.7%). In the STKA group, manipulation under anesthesia was performed in 23 subjects in 5 studies of 300 knees (range 1.3%–17.9%). McAllister and Stepanian[30] reported a significantly higher rate of manipulation in the STKA group (see **Tables 4** and **5**).

DISCUSSION

Two of the greatest concerns for patients before total joint arthroplasty are pain and length of recovery.[57] Since its introduction, MITKA has been intensively marketed. Clearly, the modern era's communications technology and sophisticated marketing techniques have dramatically influenced the speed with which new techniques are recognized, popularized, and thus demanded by an easily influenced public. However, despite the available literature on MITKA, it is important to critically review the strength of evidence before new techniques are added to the surgeon's armamentarium. The CMS[18] assesses the quality of the studies, helping to verify the methodology of the results presented.

Our review shows a mean CMS of 60 in the reported literature, suggesting that most studies reporting on outcomes of MITKA are of moderate scientific quality only. As a group, subjects who underwent MITKA tended to have decreased postoperative pain, rapid recovery of quadriceps function, reduced blood loss, improved range of motion (mostly reported as a short-term gain) and shorter hospital stay compared with subjects who underwent STKA. These benefits need to be critically balanced against the incidence of increased tourniquet time and increased incidence of component malalignment which, in turn, can lead to increased rate of implant failure[58] in the MITKA group.

The differences in positive outcomes may arise from strict subject selection criteria in the MITKA group. A subject's weight (>100 kg), body mass index (BMI >40), knee deformity (not more than

10° of anatomic varus, 15° of anatomic valgus, and a 10° flexion contracture), age (>80 years), previous open knee surgery, inflammatory arthropathy, preoperative knee range of motion (flexion <90°), and patella baja all are reported as exclusion criteria,[30,31,33,39,54,55,59,60] limiting the generalizability of these results. Also, separate anesthetic protocols and aggressive physiotherapy input in MITKA subjects may have pushed the results in its favor.[43,44] Similarly, difference in negative outcomes could be due to learning curve of the surgeons.[26,35,42]

With only four prospective randomized control trials and relatively short follow-up reported in most studies on this subject, there is a strong need for multicenter randomized controlled trials with adequate statistical power and long-term follow-up comparing MITKA with STKA.

Although there is certainly a future in MITKA, its introduction to the surgical community must be undertaken responsibly not just by the orthopedic community but also by orthopedic manufacturers. Currently, the National Institute of Clinical Excellence in England considers the evidence on the procedure's safety and efficacy inadequate for it to be undertaken without special arrangements for consent and for audit and research. It further defines the importance of training, and has asked to British Orthopaedic Association to produce standards for training.[61]

SUMMARY

Evidence-based knowledge regarding results of MITKA comes from prospective studies of moderate quality with a short follow-up period. Thus, the future of MITKA will require better visualization (eg, improved surgical approaches, whether single-incision or multi-incision), access (eg, tissue expanders, endoscopic visualization), instrumentation (ie, smaller and less bulky), and implants (eg, downsized implants with reduced fixation keels, modular implants) with longer-term follow-up studies to prove its equivalence or superiority to STKA.

REFERENCES

1. Peltier LF. The history of hip surgery. In: Callaghan JJ, Rosenberg AG, Rubash HE, editors. The adult hip. Philadelphia: Lippincott; 1998. p. 4–19.
2. Insall J, Ranawat CS, Scott WN, et al. Total condylar knee replacement: preliminary report. Clin Orthop 1976;120:149–54.
3. Insall J, Tria AJ, Scott WN. The total condylar knee prosthesis: the first five years. Clin Orthop 1979; 145:68–77.

4. Keating EM, Meding JB, Faris PM, et al. Long-term follow-up of non modular total knee replacements. Clin Orthop 2004;404:34–9.

5. Buechel FF Sr. Long-term follow up after mobile-bearing total knee replacement. Clin Orthop 2002; 403:40–50.

6. Salmon P, Hall GM, Peerbhoy D, et al. Recovery from hip and knee arthroplasty: patients perspective on pain, function, quality of life, and well-being up to 6 months postoperatively. Arch Phys Med Rehabil 2001;82:360–6.

7. Mizner RL, Petterson SC, Snyder-Mackler L. Quadriceps strength and the time course of functional recovery after total knee arthroplasty. J Orthop Sports Phys Ther 2005;35:424–36.

8. Silva M, Shepherd EF, Jackson WO, et al. Knee strength after total knee arthroplasty. J Arthroplasty 2003;18:605–11.

9. Price AJ, Webb J, Topf H, et al. Rapid recovery after Oxford unicompartmental arthroplasty through a short incision. J Arthroplasty 2001;16:970–6.

10. Argenson JN, Flecher X. Minimally invasive unicompartmental knee arthroplasty. Knee 2004;11: 341–7.

11. Rees JL, Price AJ, Breard DJ, et al. Minimally invasive Oxford unicompartmental knee arthroplasty: functional results at 1 year and the effect of surgical inexperience. Knee 2004;11:363–7.

12. Bonutti PM, Mont MA, Kester MA. Minimally invasive total knee arthroplasty: a 10-feature evolutionary approach. Orthop Clin North Am 2004;35(2):217–26.

13. Berend KR, Lombardi AV Jr. Avoiding the potential pitfalls of minimally invasive total knee surgery. Orthopedics 2005;28(11):1326–30.

14. Scuderi GR, Tenholder M, Capeci C. Surgical approaches in mini-incision total knee arthroplasty. Clin Orthop 2004;428:61–7.

15. Laskin RS. Reduced-incision total knee replacement through a mini-midvastus technique. J Knee Surg 2006;19(1):52–7.

16. Bonutti PM, Mont MA, McMahon M, et al. Minimally invasive total knee arthroplasty. J Bone Joint Surg Am 2004;86:26–32.

17. Whiteside LA. Mini incision: occasionally desirable, rarely necessary: in the affirmative. J Arthroplasty 2006;21:16–8.

18. Coleman BD, Khan KD, Maffulli N, et al. Studies of surgical outcome after patellar tendinopathy: clinical significance of methodological deficiencies and guidelines for future studies. Scand J Med Sci Sports 2000;10:2–11.

19. Tallon C, Coleman BD, Khan KM, et al. Outcome of surgery for chronic Achilles tendinopathy. A critical review. Am J Sports Med 2001;29(3):315–20.

20. Crawford R, Walley G, Bridgman S, et al. Magnetic resonance imaging versus arthroscopy in the diagnosis of knee pathology, concentrating on meniscal lesions and ACL tears: a systematic review. Br Med Bull 2007;84:5–23.

21. Mahmood A, Zafar MS, Majid I, et al. Minimally invasive hip arthroplasty: a quantitative review of the literature. Br Med Bull 2007;84:37–48.

22. Jakobsen RB, Engebretsen L, Slauterbeck JR. An analysis of the quality of cartilage repair studies. J Bone Joint Surg Am 2005;87:2232–9.

23. Moher D, Schulz KF, Altman DG. The CONSORT statement: revised recommendations for improving the quality of reports of parallel group randomized trials. BMC Med Res Methodol 2001;1:2.

24. Landis JR, Koch GG. The measurement of observer agreement for categorical data. Biometrics 1977; 33(1):59–74.

25. Shrout PE, Fleiss JL. Intraclass correlations: uses in assessing rater reliability. Psychol Bull 1979;86:420–8.

26. Tanavalee A, Thiengwittayaporn S, Itiravivong P. Progressive quadriceps incision during minimally invasive surgery for total knee arthroplasty: the effect on early postoperative ambulation. J Arthroplasty 2007;22(7):1013–8.

27. Schroer WC, Diesfeld PJ, LeMarr A, et al. Applicability of the mini-subvastus total knee arthroplasty technique: an analysis of 725 cases with mean 2-year follow-up. J Surg Orthop Adv 2007;16(3):131–7.

28. Berger RA, Sanders S, D'Ambrogio E, et al. Minimally invasive quadriceps-sparing TKA: results of a comprehensive pathway for outpatient TKA. J Knee Surg 2006;19(2):145–8.

29. Karachalios T, Giotikas D, Roidis N, et al. Total knee replacement performed with either a mini-midvastus or a standard approach: a prospective randomised clinical and radiological trial. J Bone Joint Surg Br 2008;90:584–91.

30. McAllister CM, Stepanian JD. The impact of minimally invasive surgical techniques on early range of motion after primary total knee arthroplasty. J Arthroplasty 2008;23(1):10–8.

31. Boerger TO, Aglietti P, Mondanelli N, et al. Mini-subvastus versus medial parapatellar approach in total knee arthroplasty. Clin Orthop 2005;440:82–7.

32. Laskin RS. Minimally invasive total knee arthroplasty: the results justify its use. Clin Orthop 2005; 440:54–9.

33. Huang HT, Su JY, Chang JK, et al. The early clinical outcome of minimally invasive quadriceps-sparing total knee arthroplasty: report of a 2-year follow-up. J Arthroplasty 2007;22(7):1007–12.

34. Kolisek FR, Bonutti PM, Hozack WJ, et al. Clinical experience using a minimally invasive surgical approach for total knee arthroplasty: early results of a prospective randomized study compared to a standard approach. J Arthroplasty 2007;22(1):8–13.

35. King J, Stamper DL, Schaad DC, et al. Minimally invasive total knee arthroplasty compared with traditional total knee arthroplasty. Assessment of the

learning curve and the postoperative recuperative period. J Bone Joint Surg Am 2007;89(7):1497–503.

36. Dalury DF, Dennis DA. Mini-incision total knee arthroplasty can increase risk of component malalignment. Clin Orthop 2005;440:77–81.

37. Tashiro Y, Miura H, Matsuda S, et al. Minimally invasive versus standard approach in total knee arthroplasty. Clin Orthop 2007;463:144–50.

38. Tenholder M, Clarke HD, Scuderi GR. Minimal-incision total knee arthroplasty: the early clinical experience. Clin Orthop 2005;440:67–76.

39. Laskin RS, Beksac B, Phongjunakorn A, et al. Minimally invasive total knee replacement through a mini-midvastus incision: an outcome study. Clin Orthop 2004;428:74–81.

40. Han I, Seong SC, Lee S, et al. Simultaneous bilateral MIS-TKA results in faster functional recovery. Clin Orthop 2008;466:1449–53.

41. Chotanaphuti T, Ongnamthip P, Karnchanalerk K, et al. Comparative study between 2 cm limited quadriceps exposure minimal invasive surgery and conventional total knee arthroplasty in quadriceps function: prospective randomized controlled trial. J Med Assoc Thai 2008;91(2):203–7.

42. Shankar NS. Minimally invasive technique in total knee arthroplasty—history, tips, tricks and pitfalls. Injury 2006;37:S25–30.

43. Berger RA, Sanders S, Gerlinger T, et al. Outpatient total knee arthroplasty with a minimally invasive technique. J Arthroplasty 2005;20:33–8.

44. Chen AF, Alan RK, Redziniak DE, et al. Quadriceps sparing total knee replacement. The initial experience with results at two to four years. J Bone Joint Surg Br 2006;88(11):1448–53.

45. Sanders S, Buchheit K, Deirmengian C, et al. Perioperative protocols for minimally invasive total knee arthroplasty. J Knee Surg 2006;19:129–32.

46. Scuderi GR. Preoperative planning and perioperative management for minimally invasive total knee arthroplasty. Am J Orthop 2006;35:4–6.

47. Nuelle DG, Mann K. Minimal Incision Protocols for anesthesia, pain management, and physical therapy with standard incisions in hip and knee arthroplasties: the effect on early outcomes. J Arthroplasty 2007;22:20–5.

48. Kashyap SN, van Ommeren JW. Clinical experience with less invasive surgery techniques in total knee arthroplasty: a comparative study. Knee Surg Sports Traumatol Arthrosc 2008;16(6):544–8.

49. Tria AJ Jr, Coon TM. Minimal incision total knee arthroplasty: early experience. Clin Orthop 2003; 416:185–90.

50. Haas SB, Manitta MA, Burdick P. Minimally invasive total knee arthroplasty: the mini midvastus approach. Clin Orthop 2006;452:112–6.

51. Aglietti P, Baldini A, Sensi L. Quadriceps-sparing versus mini-subvastus approach in total knee arthroplasty. Clin Orthop 2006;452:106–11.

52. Pagnano MW, Meneghini RM. Minimally invasive total knee arthroplasty with an optimized subvastus approach. J Arthroplasty 2006;21:22–6.

53. Seyler TM, Bonutti PM, Ulrich SD, et al. Minimally invasive lateral approach to total knee arthroplasty. J Arthroplasty 2007;22:21–6.

54. Bonutti PM, Neal DJ, Kester MA. Minimal incision total knee arthroplasty using the suspended leg technique. Orthopedics 2003;26(9):899–903.

55. Haas SB, Cook S, Beksac B. Minimally invasive total knee replacement through a mini midvastus approach: a comparative study. Clin Orthop 2004;428:68–73.

56. Schroer WC, Diesfeld PJ, Reedy ME, et al. Mini-subvastus approach for total knee arthroplasty. J Arthroplasty 2008;23(1):19–25.

57. Trousdale RT, McGrory BJ, Berry DJ, et al. Patients' concerns prior to undergoing total hip and total knee arthroplasty. Mayo Clin Proc 1999;74:978–82.

58. Berend ME, Ritter MA, Meding JB, et al. Tibial component failure mechanisms in total knee arthroplasty. Clin Orthop 2004;428:26–34.

59. Tria AJ Jr. Minimally invasive total knee arthroplasty: the importance of instrumentation. Orthop Clin North Am 2004;35:227–34.

60. Tria AJ Jr. Advancements in minimal invasive total knee arthroplasty. Orthopedics 2003;26:859–63.

61. Available at: www.nice.org.uk. Accessed July 20, 2008.

Minimally Invasive Surgery of the Achilles Tendon

Nicola Maffulli, MD, MS, PhD, FRCS (Orth)[a,*],
Umile Giuseppe Longo, MD[b], Francesco Oliva, MD, PhD[c],
Mario Ronga, MD[d], Vincenzo Denaro, MD[c]

KEYWORDS

- Achilles tendon • Tendinopathy • Rupture
- Minimally invasive • Percutaneous repair • Surgery

Traditional open surgical approaches for the management both of tendinopathy and ruptures of the Achilles tendon (AT) have resulted in high risk of infection and morbidity.[1] Consequently, minimally invasive surgical approaches have been developed.[2–6]

Advocates of minimally invasive AT surgery cite faster recovery times, shorter hospital stays, and improved functional outcomes as the principal reasons for adopting these new approaches when compared to traditional open techniques.[2–5] Open procedures on the AT can lead to difficulty with wound healing because of the tenuous blood supply and increased chance of wound breakdown and infection.[1] Moreover, the broad exposure given by open procedures may cause extensive iatrogenic disruption of the subcutaneous tissues and paratenon, increasing the potential for peritendinous adhesions. Critics have raised questions about increased percentage of complications (eg, sural nerve damage).

The authors present the recent advances in the field of minimally invasive AT surgery for tendinopathy, acute ruptures, and chronic tears. First we focus on our techniques of multiple percutaneous longitudinal tenotomies,[5,6] and our minimally invasive technique of stripping the AT.[2] Second, we present our method of operating on acute AT

ruptures percutaneously.[4] Last, we address the minimally invasive reconstruction of chronic tears of the AT using the peroneus brevis[3] and the semitendinous autologus tendon graft.[7]

ACHILLES TENDINOPATHY MANAGEMENT: EVOLVING CONCEPTS

The etiology of pain in Achilles tendinopathy is widely debated, with recent evidence that neovascularization and neoinnervation may be responsible.[8–14] Neovascularization is often present in patients who have tendinopathy, and the area in which patients perceive most pain correlates with the area where most neovascularization occurs on power Doppler ultrasound (US) scan.[11]

Historically, the management of Achilles tendinopathy has focused on the area of tendinopathy within the tendon. The aim of surgery was to excise fibrotic adhesions and remove degenerated nodules. Other options included producing multiple longitudinal tenotomies along the long axis of the tendon to (1) detect intratendinous lesions, (2) restore vascularity, and (3) possibly stimulate the remaining viable cells to initiate cell matrix response and healing.[15]

In patients who have isolated Achilles tendinopathy with no paratendinous involvement and

[a] Centre for Sports and Exercise Medicine, Barts and The London School of Medicine and Dentistry, Mile End Hospital, 275 Bancroft Road, London E1 4DG, UK
[b] Department of Orthopaedic and Trauma Surgery, Campus Biomedico University, Via Alvaro del Portillo, 200, 00128 Rome, Italy
[c] Department of Orthopaedics and Traumatology, University of Rome "Tor Vergata", 1, 00155 Rome, Italy
[d] Department of Orthopaedic and Trauma Surgery, University of Insubria, Via di Circolo, 1, Varese, Italy
* Corresponding author.
E-mail address: n.maffulli@qmul.ac.uk (N. Maffulli).

Orthop Clin N Am 40 (2009) 491–498
doi:10.1016/j.ocl.2009.05.006
0030-5898/09/$ – see front matter © 2009 Elsevier Inc. All rights reserved.

a well-defined nodular lesion less than 2.5 cm long, multiple percutaneous longitudinal tenotomies can be used when conservative management has failed.[5] A US scan may be helpful to accurately determine the precise location of tendinopathy.[6]

New surgical management options are aimed at managing the neovascularization outside the tendon.[2] To this aim, we have developed a new minimally invasive stripping of the AT.

MULTIPLE PERCUTANEOUS LONGITUDINAL TENOTOMIES

The patient lies prone on the operating table with the feet protruding beyond the edge and the ankles resting on a padded sandbag.[5] The tendon is carefully palpated, and the area of maximum swelling and/or tenderness is marked and rechecked by US scan. The skin and the subcutaneous tissues over the AT are infiltrated with 10 to 15 mL of plain 1% Lignocaine (Lignocaine Hydrochloride, Evans Medical Ltd., Leatherhead, England).

A #11 surgical scalpel blade is inserted parallel to the long axis of the tendon fibers in the marked areas with the cutting edge pointing cranially. This initial stab incision is made in the central portion of the diseased tendon. With the blade held still, a full passive ankle dorsiflexion movement is produced. After the position of the blade is reversed, a full passive ankle plantarflexion movement is produced. A tenotomy is thereby produced over a length of up to approximately 3 cm using only a stab incision. The procedure is repeated 2 cm medial and proximally, medial and distally, lateral and proximally, and lateral and distally to the site of the first stab wound. The pattern of the five stab incisions is similar to the number 5 on a die. The five wounds are closed with Steri-Strips (3M Surgical Products, St. Paul, Minnesota), dressed with cotton swabs, and several layers of cotton wool and a crepe bandage are applied.

ULTRASOUND-GUIDED PERCUTANEOUS TENOTOMY

The patient is positioned as described for the previous technique. A bloodless field is not necessary. The tendon is carefully palpated, and the area of maximum swelling and/or tenderness is marked and checked by US scan.[6] The skin is prepped with an antiseptic solution, and a sterile longitudinal 7.5 MHz US probe is used to confirm the area of tendinopathy. Before the skin and subcutaneous tissues over the AT are infiltrated with 10 mL of 1% Carbocaina (Pierrel, Milan, Italy), 7 mL of 0.5% Carbocaina is used to infiltrate the space between the tendon and the paratenon.

This brisement procedure attempts to free the paratenon from the tendon by disrupting adhesions between the two structures.

Under US guidance, a #11 surgical scalpel blade (Swann-Morton Ltd., Sheffield, England) is inserted parallel to the long axis of the tendon fibers in the center of the area of tendinopathy, as assessed by high-resolution US imaging. The cutting edge of the blade points caudally and penetrates the entire thickness of the tendon. With the blade held still, a full passive ankle flexion is produced.

All subsequent tenotomies are performed through this same stab incision unless there is an extensive area of tendinosis or an additional area of tendon disease. The scalpel blade is then retracted to the surface of the tendon inclined 45 degrees on the sagittal axis, and the blade is inserted medially through the original tenotomy. With the blade held still, a full passive ankle flexion is produced. The whole procedure is then repeated with the blade inclined 45 degrees laterally to the original tenotomy and inserted laterally through the original tenotomy. Again with the blade kept still, a full passive ankle flexion is produced. The blade is then partially retracted to the posterior surface of the AT, reversed 180 degrees so that its cutting edge now points cranially, and the procedure is repeated, with care taken to dorsiflex the ankle passively. Preliminary cadaveric studies demonstrated that, on average, a 2.8-cm tenotomy is obtained using this technique. The stab wound can be dressed with a Steri-Strip, or left open.[16,17] The wound is dressed with cotton swabs, and several layers of cotton wool and a crepe bandage are applied.

MINIMALLY INVASIVE STRIPPING

The patient undergoes local or general anesthesia, according to surgeon or patient preference. The patient is positioned prone with a calf tourniquet, which is inflated to 250 mmHg after exsanguination. Skin preparation is performed in the usual fashion.

Four skin incisions are made. The first two are 0.5-cm longitudinal incisions at the proximal origin of the AT, just medial and lateral to the origin of the tendon. The other two incisions are also 0.5 cm long and longitudinal, but 1 cm distal to the distal end of the tendon insertion on the calcaneus.

A mosquito clamp is inserted in the proximal incisions, and the AT is freed of the peritendinous adhesions. A #1 unmounted Ethibond (Ethicon, Somerville, New Jersey) suture thread is inserted proximally, passing through the two proximal incisions. The thread is retrieved from the distal incisions, over the posterior aspect of the AT.

Using a gentle seesaw motion, similar to using a Gigli saw, the Ethibond suture thread is made to slide posterior to the tendon, which is stripped and freed from Kager's triangle.

The procedure is repeated for the posterior aspect of the AT. If necessary, using a #11 blade, longitudinal percutaneous tenotomies parallel to the tendon fibers are made.[5,6,18]

The subcutaneous and subcuticular tissues are closed in a routine fashion, and Mepore (Mölnlycke Health Care, Gothenburg, Sweden) dressings are applied to the skin. A removable Scotchcast (St. Paul, Minnesota; Smith & Nephew, Inc., Charlotte, North Carolina) support with Velcro straps can be applied if deemed necessary.

POSTOPERATIVE CARE

Postoperatively, patients are allowed mobilization with full weight bearing. After 2 weeks, the cast, if used, is removed, and physiotherapy is begun, focusing on proprioception, plantar flexion of the ankle, inversion, and eversion.

ACUTE ACHILLES TENDON RUPTURE

The AT is the most commonly ruptured tendon in the human body.[3,19] The management of acutely ruptured AT largely depends on the preference of the surgeon or the patient. Management can be broadly classified into operative (ie, open or percutaneous) and nonoperative (eg, cast immobilization or functional bracing).[20] The management of AT ruptures has changed with time, as more evidence supports early mobilization[21–23] and the use of percutaneous techniques instead of open surgery. Recent systematic reviews have shown that open operative management of acute AT ruptures significantly reduces the risk of rerupture compared with nonoperative treatment, as it allows accurate apposition of the ruptured tendon ends and earlier motion. However, operative management is associated with a significantly higher risk of wound-healing problems.[1] Operative risks may be reduced by performing surgery percutaneously.[20,24]

The goals of managing AT ruptures are to minimize the morbidity of the injury, optimize rapid return to full function, and prevent complications. Ismail and colleagues[25] recently reported on the Achillon mini-incision technique, comparing the basic mechanical properties of the tendon suture performed using the Achillon method with those of the long-established Kessler method, and assessing whether the strength of the repair was related to tendon diameter. They conclude that the Achillon repair had comparable tensile strength to the Kessler repair.

The authors prefer Carmont and Maffulli's technique[4] in comparison with the Achillon repair: the first procedure is less expensive, and promotes a stronger repair, as it allows the use of a greater number of suture strands (eight) for the repair of the AT. Biomechanical studies are ongoing, and preliminary results seem to validate our opinion.

PERCUTANEOUS REPAIR OF ACUTE ACHILLES TENDON RUPTURE

The patient is positioned prone. Areas 4–6 cm proximal and distal to the palpable tendon defect and the skin over the defect are infiltrated with 20 mL of 1% Lignocaine. Ten ml of Chirocaine 0.5% (Purdue Pharma, Stamford, Connecticut) are infiltrated deep into the tendon defect. A calf tourniquet, skin preparation, and steridrapes are applied.

A 1 cm transverse incision is made over the defect using a #11 blade. Four longitudinal stab incisions are made lateral and medial to the tendon 6 cm proximal to the palpable defect. Two further longitudinal incisions on either side of the tendon are made 4–6 cm distal to the palpable defect. Forceps are then used to mobilize the tendon from beneath the subcutaneous tissues. A 9 cm Mayo needle (BL059N, #B00 round point spring eye, B Braun, Aesculap, Tuttlingen, Germany) is threaded with two double loops of #1 Maxon (Tyco Healthcare, Norwalk, Connecticut), and this is passed transversely between the proximal stab incisions through the bulk of the tendon. The bulk of the tendon is surprisingly superficial. The loose ends are held with a clip. In turn, each of the ends is then passed distally from just proximal to the transverse Maxon passage through the bulk of the tendon to pass through the diagonally opposing stab incision. A subsequent diagonal pass is then made to the transverse incision over the ruptured tendon. To prevent entanglement, both ends of the Maxon are held in separate clips. This suture is then tested for security by pulling distally with both ends of the Maxon. Another double loop of Maxon is then passed between the distal stabs incisions through the tendon, and, in turn, through the tendon and out of the transverse incision starting distal to the transverse passage. The ankle is held in full plantar flexion, and, in turn, opposing ends of the Maxon thread are tied together with a double throw knot, and then three further throws before being buried using the forceps. A clip is used to hold the first throw of the lateral side to maintain the tension of the suture.

A subcuticular Biosyn suture 3.0 (Tyco Healthcare) is used to close the transverse incision, and Steri-Strips are applied to the stab incisions.

Finally, a Mepore dressing is applied, and a bivalved removable Scotchcast in full plantar flexion is applied and held in place with Velcro straps.

The patient is allowed to return home on the day of surgery, and can bear full weight as able in the cast in full plantar flexion. At 2 weeks, the wounds are inspected, and the back shell of the cast is removed, allowing proprioception, plantar flexion, inversion, and eversion exercises. The front shell remains in place for 6 weeks to prevent forced dorsiflexion of the ankle.

CHRONIC ACHILLES TENDON RUPTURES

The management of chronic AT ruptures is usually different from that of acute rupture, as the tendon ends normally will have retracted.[3,26,27] The blood supply to this area is relatively poor, and the tendon ends have to be freshened to allow healing. Due to the increased gap, primary repair is not generally possible.[27] Operative procedures for reconstruction of the AT include flap tissue turn-down using one[28,29] and two flaps,[30] local tendon transfer,[31-34] and autologous hamstring tendon harvesting.[35] All of these techniques use a single longitudinal incision for exposure. Following these procedures, complications, especially wound breakdown and infection,[36] are not infrequent, are probably related to the paucity of the soft tissue vascularity, and may require plastic surgical procedures to cover significant soft tissue defects.[37]

We have recently described a less invasive technique of peroneus brevis reconstruction for the AT using two paramidline incisions.[3] This technique allows reconstruction of the AT using peroneus brevis, thus preserving skin integrity over the site most prone to wound breakdown. During surgery, after trying to reduce the gap of the ruptured AT, the resulting gap is sometimes greater than 6 cm despite maximal plantar flexion of the ankle and traction on the AT stumps.[3] In such instances, peroneus brevis is not sufficient to fill the gap; an alternative is to harvest the ipsilateral hamstring tendon, described below.[34]

PERONEUS BREVIS TRANSFER

The patient is positioned prone with a calf tourniquet. Skin preparation is performed in the usual fashion, and sterile drapes are applied. Preoperative anatomical markings include the palpable tendon defect, both malleoli, and the base of the fifth metatarsal.

Three skin incisions are made, and accurate hemostasis by ligation of the larger veins and diathermy of the smaller ones is performed.[3] The first incision is a 5-cm longitudinal incision, made 2 cm proximal and just medial to the palpable end of the residual tendon. The second incision is 3 cm long and also longitudinal but is 2 cm distal and lateral to the distal end of the tendon rupture. Care is taken to prevent damage to the sural nerve by making this incision as close as possible to the anterior aspect of the lateral border of the AT to avoid the nerve. At the level of the AT insertion, the sural nerve is 18.8 mm lateral to the tendon but, as it progresses proximally, the nerve gradually traverses medially crossing the lateral border of the tendon 9.8 cm proximal to the calcaneus. Thus, the second incision avoids the sural nerve by being placed on the lateral side of the AT but medial to the nerve. The third incision is a 2-cm longitudinal incision at the base of the fifth metatarsal.

The distal AT stump is mobilized, freeing it of all the peritendinous adhesions, particularly on the lateral aspect. This allows access to the base of the lateral aspect of the distal tendon close to its insertion. It should be possible to palpate the medial tubercle of the calcaneus. The ruptured tendon end is then resected back to healthy tendon, and a #1 Vicryl (Ethicon Inc., Somerville, New Jersey) locking suture is run along the free tendon edge to prevent separation of the bundles.

The proximal tendon is then mobilized from the proximal wound, any adhesions are divided, and further soft tissue release anterior to the soleus and gastrocnemius allows maximal excursion, minimizing the gap between the two tendon stumps. A Vicryl locking suture is run along the free tendon edge to allow adequate exposure and to prevent separation of the bundles.

The tendon of peroneus brevis is harvested. The tendon is identified through the incision on the lateral border of the foot at its insertion at the base of the fifth metatarsal. The tendon is exposed, and a #1 Vicryl locking suture is applied to the tendon end before release from the metatarsal base. The tendon of peroneus brevis is identified at the base of the distal incision of the AT following incision of the deep fascia overlying the peroneal muscles compartment. The tendon of peroneus brevis is then withdrawn through the distal wound. This may take significant force, as there may be tendinous strands between the two peroneal tendons distally. The muscular portion of peroneus brevis is then mobilized proximally to allow increased excursion of the tendon of peroneus brevis.

A longitudinal tenotomy parallel to the tendon fibers is made through both stumps of the tendon. A clip is used to develop the plane, from lateral to medial, in the distal stump of the AT, and the peroneus brevis graft is passed through the tenotomy. With the ankle in maximal plantar flexion, a #1 Vicryl suture is used to suture the peroneus brevis to both sides of the distal stump. The tendon of peroneus brevis is then passed beneath the intact skin bridge into the proximal incision, and passed from medial to lateral through a transverse tenotomy in the proximal stump, and further secured with #1 Vicryl. Finally, the tendon of peroneus brevis is sutured back onto itself on the lateral side of the proximal incision. The reconstruction may be further augmented using a Maxon suture.

The wounds are closed with 2.0 Vicryl, 3.0 Biosyn, and Steri-Strips, taking care to avoid the risk of postoperative hematoma and minimize wound breakdown. A previously prepared removable Scotchcast support with Velcro straps is applied.

Postoperatively, patients are allowed to bear weight as comfort allows with the use of elbow crutches. After 2 weeks, the back shell of the cast is removed, and physiotherapy is begun with the front shell in situ to prevent dorsiflexion of the ankle, focusing on proprioception, plantar flexion of the ankle, inversion, and eversion. During this period of rehabilitation, patients are permitted to bear weight as comfort allows with the front shell in situ, although full weight bearing rarely occurs on account of balance difficulties and patients usually still require the assistance of a single elbow crutch as this stage. The front shell may be removed after 6 weeks. The authors do not use a heel raise after removal of the cast, and patients normally regain a plantigrade ankle over a couple of weeks.

IPSILATERAL FREE SEMITENDINOSUS TENDON GRAFT TRANSFER FOR CHRONIC TEARS OF THE ACHILLES TENDON

The patient is positioned prone with a calf tourniquet. Skin preparation is performed in the usual fashion, and sterile drapes are applied. Preoperative anatomical markings include the palpable tendon defect and both malleoli.[7] Two skin incisions are made (Fig. 1), and accurate hemostasis by ligation of the larger veins and diathermy of the smaller ones is performed. The first incision is a 5-cm longitudinal incision, made 2 cm proximal and just medial to the palpable end of the residual tendon. The second incision is 3 cm long and is also longitudinal, but is 2 cm distal and in the midline over the distal end of the tendon rupture. Care is taken to prevent damage to the sural nerve. At the level of the AT insertion, the sural nerve is 18.8 mm lateral to the tendon but, as it progresses proximally, the nerve gradually

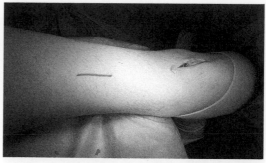

Fig. 1. Two skin incisions are made. The first incision is a 5-cm longitudinal incision, made 2 cm proximal and just medial to the palpable end of the residual tendon. The second incision is 3 cm long and is also longitudinal but is 2 cm distal and in the midline over the distal end of the tendon rupture.

traverses medially, crossing the lateral border of the tendon 9.8 cm proximal to the calcaneus.[38] Thus, the second incision avoids the sural nerve by being placed medial to the nerve.

The proximal and distal AT stump are mobilized, freeing them of all the peritendinous adhesions (Figs. 2 and 3). It should be possible to palpate the medial tubercle of the calcaneus. The ruptured tendon end is then resected back to healthy tendon, and a #1 Vicryl locking suture is run along the free tendon edge to prevent separation of the bundles (Fig. 4).

The proximal tendon is then mobilized from the proximal wound, any adhesions are divided, and further soft tissue release anterior to the soleus and gastrocnemius allows maximal excursion, minimizing the gap between the two tendon stumps. A Vicryl locking suture is run along the free tendon edge to allow adequate exposure and to prevent separation of the bundles.

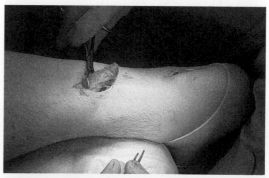

Fig. 2. The proximal AT stump is mobilized, freeing it of all peritendinous adhesions. The ruptured tendon end is then resected back to healthy tendon.

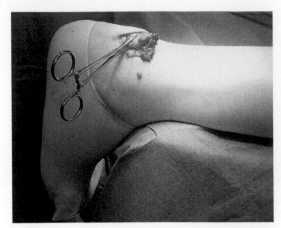

Fig. 3. The distal AT stump is mobilized, freeing it of all peritendinous adhesions. The ruptured tendon end is then resected back to healthy tendon.

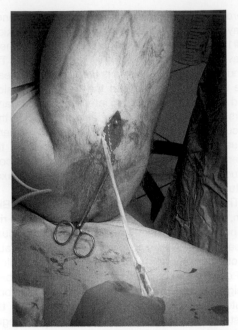

Fig. 5. The tendon of the semitendinosus is harvested through a vertical, 2.5–3 cm longitudinal incision over the pes anserinus.

After trying to reduce the gap of the ruptured AT, if the gap produced is greater than 6 cm despite maximal plantar flexion of the ankle and traction on the AT stumps, the ipsilateral semitendinosus is harvested.

The tendon of the semitendinosus is harvested through a vertical, 2.5–3 cm longitudinal incision over the pes anserinus (**Fig. 5**). The semitendinosus tendon is passed through a small incision in the substance of the proximal stump of the AT (**Fig. 6**), and it is sutured to the AT at the entry and exit points using 3-0 Vicryl (Polyglactin 910 braided absorbable suture; Johnson & Johnson, Brussels, Belgium). The semitendinosus tendon is then passed beneath the intact skin bridge into the distal incision, and passed from medial to lateral through a transverse tenotomy in the distal stump. With the ankle in maximal plantar flexion,

the semitendinosus tendon is sutured to the AT at each entry and exit point using 3-0 Vicryl. The repair is tensioned to maximal equinus.

One extremity of the semitendinosus tendon is then passed again beneath the intact skin bridge into the proximal incision, and passed from medial to lateral through a transverse tenotomy in the proximal stump. The other extremity of the semitendinosus tendon is then passed again from medial to lateral through a transverse tenotomy in the distal stump. The reconstruction may be further augmented using a Maxon suture (**Fig. 7**). The

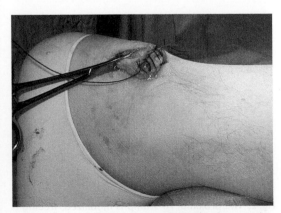

Fig. 4. A locking suture is run along the free tendon edge to prevent separation of the bundles.

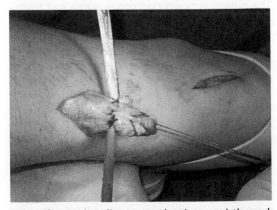

Fig. 6. The semitendinosus tendon is passed through a small incision in the substance of the proximal stump of the AT.

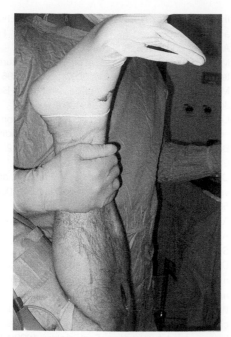

Fig. 7. The final result.

wounds are closed with 2.0 Vicryl, 3,0 Biosyn, and Steri-Strips. A previously prepared removable Scotchcast support with Velcro straps is applied.

Postoperatively, patients are allowed to bear weight as comfort allows with the use of elbow crutches.[21,22] After 2 weeks, the back shell of the cast is removed, and physiotherapy is begun with the front shell in situ preventing dorsiflexion of the ankle, focusing on proprioception, plantar flexion of the ankle, inversion, and eversion.[21,22] During this period of rehabilitation, patients are permitted to bear weight as comfort allows with the front shell in situ, although full weight bearing rarely occurs on account of balance difficulties and patients usually still require the assistance of a single elbow crutch as this stage. The front shell may be removed after 0 weeks. The authors do not use a heel raise after removal of the cast, and patients normally regain a plantigrade ankle over 2 to 3 weeks.[21,22]

SUMMARY

The nascent literature on minimally invasive AT surgery is far from universally supportive. Most series that have been published in support of these surgical approaches are first reports by originators of particular techniques. Randomized controlled trials are required to address the issue of the comparison between open versus minimally invasive AT surgery. In the authors' experience, minimally invasive surgery has provided similar results to those obtained with open surgery, in addition to providing decreased perioperative morbidity, decreased duration of hospital stay, and reduced costs. All the minimally invasive techniques described in this article are inexpensive, and they do not require highly specialized equipment and training.

REFERENCES

1. Saxena A, Maffulli N, Nguyen A, et al. Wound complications from surgeries pertaining to the Achilles tendon: an analysis of 219 surgeries. J Am Podiatr Med Assoc 2008;98(2):95–101.
2. Longo UG, Ramamurthy C, Denaro V, et al. Minimally invasive stripping for chronic Achilles tendinopathy. Disabil Rehabil 2008;30(20–2):1709–13.
3. Carmont MR, Maffulli N. Less invasive Achilles tendon reconstruction. BMC Musculoskelet Disord 2007;8:100.
4. Carmont MR, Maffulli N. Modified percutaneous repair of ruptured Achilles tendon. Knee Surg Sports Traumatol Arthrosc 2008;16(2):199–203.
5. Maffulli N, Testa V, Capasso G, et al. Results of percutaneous longitudinal tenotomy for Achilles tendinopathy in middle- and long-distance runners. Am J Sports Med 1997;25(6):835–40.
6. Testa V, Capasso G, Benazzo F, et al. Management of Achilles tendinopathy by ultrasound-guided percutaneous tenotomy. Med Sci Sports Exerc 2002;34(4):573–80.
7. Maffulli N, Longo UG, Gougoulias N, et al. Ipsilateral free semitendinosus tendon graft transfer for reconstruction of chronic tears of the Achilles tendon. BMC Musculoskelet Disord 2008;9:100.
8. Alfredson H, Ohberg L, Forsgren S. Is vasculoneural ingrowth the cause of pain in chronic Achilles tendinosis? An investigation using ultrasonography and colour Doppler, immunohistochemistry, and diagnostic injections. Knee Surg Sports Traumatol Arthrosc 2003;11(5):334–8,
9. Knobloch K, Kraemer R, Lichtenberg A, et al. Achilles tendon and paratendon microcirculation in midportion and insertional tendinopathy in athletes. Am J Sports Med 2006;34(1):92–7.
10. Kristoffersen M, Ohberg L, Johnston C, et al. Neovascularisation in chronic tendon injuries detected with colour Doppler ultrasound in horse and man: implications for research and treatment. Knee Surg Sports Traumatol Arthrosc 2005;13(6):505–8.
11. Ohberg L, Lorentzon R, Alfredson H. Neovascularisation in Achilles tendons with painful tendinosis but not in normal tendons: an ultrasonographic investigation. Knee Surg Sports Traumatol Arthrosc 2001;9(4):233–8.
12. Maffulli N, Sharma P, Luscombe KL. Achilles tendinopathy: aetiology and management. J R Soc Med 2004;97(10):472–6.

13. Maffulli N, Testa V, Capasso G, et al. Similar histopathological picture in males with Achilles and patellar tendinopathy. Med Sci Sports Exerc 2004; 36(9):1470–5.

14. Maffulli N, Wong J, Almekinders LC. Types and epidemiology of tendinopathy. Clin Sports Med 2003;22(4):675–92.

15. Rolf C, Movin T. Etiology, histopathology, and outcome of surgery in achillodynia. Foot Ankle Int 1997;18(9):565–9.

16. Maffulli N, Pintore E, Petricciuolo F. Arthroscopy wounds: to suture or not to suture. Acta Orthop Belg 1991;57(2):154–6.

17. Maffulli N, Dymond NP, Regine R. Surgical repair of ruptured Achilles tendon in sportsmen and sedentary patients: a longitudinal ultrasound assessment. Int J Sports Med 1990;11(1):78–84.

18. Sayana MK, Maffulli N. Eccentric calf muscle training in non-athletic patients with Achilles tendinopathy. J Sci Med Sport 2007;10(1):52–8.

19. Ames PR, Longo UG, Denaro V, et al. Achilles tendon problems: not just an orthopaedic issue. Disabil Rehabil 2008;30(20–22):1646–50.

20. Ebinesan AD, Sarai BS, Walley GD, et al. Conservative, open or percutaneous repair for acute rupture of the Achilles tendon. Disabil Rehabil 2008;30(20–22):1721–5.

21. Maffulli N, Tallon C, Wong J, et al. Early weightbearing and ankle mobilization after open repair of acute midsubstance tears of the Achilles tendon. Am J Sports Med 2003;31(5):692–700.

22. Maffulli N, Tallon C, Wong J, et al. No adverse effect of early weight bearing following open repair of acute tears of the Achilles tendon. J Sports Med Phys Fitness 2003;43(3):367–79.

23. Maffulli N. Immediate weight-bearing is not detrimental to operatively or conservatively managed rupture of the Achilles tendon. Aust J Physiother 2006;52:225.

24. Khan RJ, Fick D, Keogh A, et al. Treatment of acute Achilles tendon ruptures. A meta-analysis of randomized, controlled trials. J Bone Joint Surg Am 2005;87(10):2202–10.

25. Ismail M, Karim A, Shulman R, et al. The Achillon achilles tendon repair: is it strong enough? Foot Ankle Int 2008;29(8):808–13.

26. Maffulli N, Ajis A, Longo UG, et al. Chronic rupture of tendo Achillis. Foot Ankle Clin 2007;12(4):583–96, vi.

27. Maffulli N. Rupture of the Achilles tendon. J Bone Joint Surg Am 1999;81(7):1019–36.

28. Lee YS, Lin CC, Chen CN, et al. Reconstruction for neglected Achilles tendon rupture: the modified Bosworth technique. Orthopedics 2005;28(7): 647–50.

29. Christensen I. Rupture of the Achilles tendon; analysis of 57 cases. Acta Chir Scand 1953;106(1): 50–60.

30. Arner O, Lindholm A. Subcutaneous rupture of the Achilles tendon; a study of 92 cases. Acta Chir Scand Suppl 1959;116(Suppl 239):1–51.

31. Dekker M, Bender J. Results of surgical treatment of rupture of the Achilles tendon with use of the plantaris tendon. Arch Chir Neerl 1977;29(1):39–46.

32. Wapner KL, Pavlock GS, Hecht PJ, et al. Repair of chronic Achilles tendon rupture with flexor hallucis longus tendon transfer. Foot Ankle 1993;14(8): 443–9.

33. Wilcox DK, Bohay DR, Anderson JG. Treatment of chronic Achilles tendon disorders with flexor hallucis longus tendon transfer/augmentation. Foot Ankle Int 2000;21(12):1004–10.

34. McClelland D, Maffulli N. Neglected rupture of the Achilles tendon: reconstruction with peroneus brevis tendon transfer. Surgeon 2004;2(4):209–13.

35. Maffulli N, Leadbetter WB. Free gracilis tendon graft in neglected tears of the Achilles tendon. Clin J Sport Med 2005;15(2):56–61.

36. Pintore E, Barra V, Pintore R, et al. Peroneus brevis tendon transfer in neglected tears of the Achilles tendon. J Trauma 2001;50(1):71–8.

37. Kumta SM, Maffulli N. Local flap coverage for soft tissue defects following open repair of Achilles tendon rupture. Acta Orthop Belg 2003;69(1):59–66.

38. Webb J, Moorjani N, Radford M. Anatomy of the sural nerve and its relation to the Achilles tendon. Foot Ankle Int 2000;21(6):475–7.

Minimally Invasive Osteosynthesis of Distal Tibial Fractures Using Locking Plates

Mario Ronga, MD[a], Chezhiyan Shanmugam, MD[b],
Umile Giuseppe Longo, MD[c], Francesco Oliva, MD, PhD[d],
Nicola Maffulli, MD, MS, PhD, FRCS (Orth)[e,*]

KEYWORDS

- Locking plates • Minimally invasive plate osteosynthesis
- Percutaneous • Distal tibial fractures
- Tibial plafond fractures • Tibial pylon fractures

Surgical fixation of distal tibia fractures can be difficult and requires careful preoperative planning. Fracture pattern, soft tissue injury, and bone quality critically influence the selection of fixation technique.[1] Several surgical methods have been described for the treatment of these fractures, including external fixation, intramedullary nailing, and plate fixation. Classic open reduction and internal plate fixation require extensive soft tissue dissection and periosteal stripping even in expert hands, with high rates of complications, including infection, delayed union, and nonunion.[2,3] Several minimally invasive plate osteosynthesis techniques have been developed, with good results at medium-term follow-up.[4–6] These techniques aim to reduce surgical trauma and to maintain a more biologically favorable environment for fracture healing.

A new advance in this field is represented by the locking plate (LP). These devices consist of plate and screw systems, wherein the screws are locked in the plate at a fixed angle. Preliminary clinical studies report a high success rate of the minimally invasive LP technique in distal tibia fractures.[7–9]

TREATMENT CONSIDERATIONS

The optimal management of distal tibial fractures remains controversial. External fixation may result in inaccurate reduction, malunion or nonunion, and pin tract infection.[10] Intramedullary nailing is considered the standard method for surgically managing diaphyseal fractures of the tibia, but the distal tibia poses concerns regarding the stability of fixation, the risk for secondary displacement of the fracture on insertion of the nail,

Each author certifies that he or she has no commercial associations (eg, consultancies, stock ownership, equity interest, patent/licensing arrangements) that might pose a conflict of interest in connection with the submitted article.

[a] Department of Orthopaedic and Trauma Surgery, University of Insubria, Ospedale di Circolo, Viale L. Borri 57, 21100 Varese, Italy

[b] Department of Trauma and Orthopaedic Surgery, Keele University School of Medicine, North Staffordshire Hospital, Thornburrow Drive, Hartshill, Stoke on Trent, Staffordshire, ST4 7QB, England, UK

[c] Department of Orthopaedic and Trauma Surgery, Campus Biomedico University, Via Longoni, 83, 00155 Rome, Italy

[d] Department of Orthopaedics and Traumatology, University of Rome "Tor Vergata" School of Medicine, Viale Oxford 81, 00133 Rome, Italy

[e] Centre for Sports and Exercise Medicine, Barts and The London School of Medicine and Dentistry, Mile End Hospital, 275 Bancroft Road, London E1 4DG, England, UK

* Corresponding author.

E-mail address: n.maffulli@qmul.ac.uk (N. Maffulli).

Orthop Clin N Am 40 (2009) 499–504
doi:10.1016/j.ocl.2009.05.007
0030-5898/09/$ – see front matter © 2009 Elsevier Inc. All rights reserved.

orthopedic.theclinics.com

breakage of nails and locking screws, and final alignment of the tibia.[11,12]

A recent meta-analysis reviewed the outcomes of different methods of management of extra-articular distal tibia fractures, comparing the rates of nonunion, infection, malunion, and secondary surgical procedures.[13] No method was superior to another, but most of the identified studies were case series and were limited by the lack of adequate control groups. The results were potentially biased by the different indications for the different surgical approaches. No studies compared external fixation with other methods, whereas one prospective[14] and three retrospective studies[12,15,16] compared plate and screws inserted through a traditional open approach with nails for the treatment of these fractures. The first study used anatomic plates, whereas the others used dynamic compression plates. The prospective study[14] and two of the three retrospective studies[15,16] did not report different rates of nonunion. They were underpowered to detect a difference, however. The prospective randomized study on 64 consecutive patients reported shorter operative times ($P = .02$), reduced wound problems ($P = .03$), and a lesser decrease of range of motion ($P = .001$) in patients treated with nails. In the plate group, the average angulation was $0.9°$ compared with $2.8°$ in the nail group ($P = .01$).[14]

Vallier and colleagues[12] reported the largest comparative series (113 fractures) consisting of 76 nails and 37 plates. The two groups were matched in terms of patient age, mechanism of injury, and fracture characteristics. Considering all patients with delayed unions or nonunions, there was a trend toward deficient healing after nailing (12% versus 2.7%; $P = .10$). Malunions were more common after intramedullary nailing (29%) versus a plate (5.4%) ($P = .003$). This could result from a selection bias of fractures with more severe soft tissue damage and comminution in the nail group. The study was limited by its retrospective nature and nonrandomized design. All studies considered evidenced that nail treatment resulted in a greater rate of malalignment compared with plate treatment.

Minimally invasive plating techniques reduce iatrogenic soft tissue injury and damage to bone vascularity, in addition to preserving the osteogenic fracture hematoma. Initial clinical series using these methods for distal tibia fractures demonstrated favorable results with low rates of infection and nonunion.[5,6,17,18] Several complications, such as angular deformities greater than $7°$, metalwork failure, and nonunions, have been reported.[4–6]

RATIONALE OF LOCKING PLATE

LPs refer to the fact that the screw heads are threaded and, when tightened, lock into threads in the plate. Thereby, a fixed-angle construct is created. Such constructs are much less prone to loosening or toggle than traditional non-LPs.[19] The precise anatomic shape of LPs prevents primary dislocation of the fracture caused by inexact contouring of a normal plate and allows a better distribution of the angular and axial loading around the plate.[20,21]

Minimally invasive surgery using LPs uses indirect reduction and maintains alignment by bridging the fracture without compression. Percutaneous plating maintains arterial vascularity by preserving the soft tissue envelope and periosteum, and thereby minimizes the surgical trauma. Moreover, screw locking minimizes the compressive forces exerted by the plate on the bone, and thus avoids disturbance of the bone blood supply.[20,21] Osteogenesis requires an adequate blood supply, and preosseous tissue can be diverted down a chondrogenic pathway in regions of low oxygen tension. For this goal, the shape of the LP minimizes the compressive forces exerted by the plate on the bone so as to avoid disturbance of the bone blood supply.[20,21]

LPs are best described as "internally placed external fixators" or "locked internal fixators;" this construct converts axial load into compression force rather than shear force as in dynamic compression plates. The system works as flexible elastic fixation that stimulates callus formation.[22] Based on the evidence that bone continuity after a fracture can be restored by primary and secondary healing,[23] some flexibility is desirable in the final fixation to stimulate callus formation and secondary bone healing. Low fracture strain results in minimal to no callus formation and primary bone healing. As the fracture strain increases, secondary healing or callus formation occurs.[24] Strain between 10% and 30% would result in bone resorption and nonunion, however.[25]

Such factors as bone contact, working length or distance of the first screw to the fracture, number of screws, and distance of the plate from the bone all contribute to rigidity of the construct. In one biomechanical test, leaving one screw hole open on either side of a fracture resulted in doubling of the flexibility of the construct in compression and torsion.[26]

For all these properties, an LP is a superior device having a biomechanical edge over a conventional plate in elderly, osteopenic, and metaphyseal bone and in highly comminuted fractures.

SURGICAL TECHNIQUE

Depending on the skin condition, surgery has to be planned when the ankle swelling has subsided and the "wrinkle sign" is present. In the wrinkle sign, the ankle is dorsiflexed while the anterior aspect of the ankle is observed; the absence of a skin crease or wrinkle suggests severe swelling.[27] Temporary skeletal stabilization can be achieved by simple splintage or bridging external fixation until surgery is performed.

Good-quality plain radiographs (anteroposterior, lateral, and long-leg alignment views) are obtained with CT scans, if necessary, to determine optimal plate location. Identification of the size and location of the articular fragments is essential before reconstruction. In the distal tibia, the plate is normally applied on the anteromedial aspect. Several precontoured plates specifically designed for these locations are commercially available. Anatomic LPs should not be bent because bending alters the biomechanical properties of the plate, possibly leading to fatigue failure.[28]

With the patient positioned supine on a radiolucent table, antibiotic prophylaxis is administered and standard intraoperative fluoroscopy is used throughout the procedure. Great care should be taken to ensure that the fracture can be clearly visualized on anteroposterior and lateral views. The injured limb and the noninjured limb are prepared and draped above the knee, thus allowing intraoperative alignment to be checked against the normal limb. Elevating the injured limb on radiolucent trays enables a clear lateral view and avoids interference from the other leg. The joint lines of the knee and the ankle are defined and marked on the skin. Using manual traction, or through a single Steinman pin inserted into the calcaneus, the fracture is reduced (**Fig. 1**). Depending on the quality of tibial fracture reduction reached, a fibula fracture, if present, can be plated first using a one-third tubular plate to provide lateral stability and restoration of the correct length and to prevent overdistraction at the fracture site. The main fracture fragments of the distal tibia are aligned and reduced percutaneously or through separate stab incisions and are then fixed with individual lag screws.

In the fractures with intra-articular extension, arthroscopy can be performed through conventional anterior portals to assess the reduction of the articular surface and to address any associated joint lesions. Several researchers reported an incidence of intra-articular pathologic findings in ankle fractures ranging between 63% and 79.2%.[29–31] Based on the minimal added time and morbidity to the surgical procedure, the

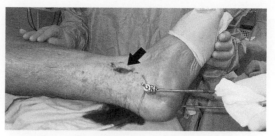

Fig. 1. Calcaneal Steinman pin and connection to a traction device. In this way, traction can be applied to reduce the fracture and maintain the length and alignment of the limb while the LP is inserted. Note the small incision distal to the medial malleolus (*arrow*).

authors use arthroscopy on a regular basis but limit its use to intra-articular fractures.

With the fracture adequately reduced, an adequate transverse incision is made distal to the medial malleolus and a subcutaneous tunnel is created (**Fig. 2**). An LP is then passed along the tunnel, bridging the fracture site. The plate has to be long enough to bridge the metaphyseal zone and to allow at least two bicortical screws insertions proximal to the fracture. Kirschner wires can be used to secure, through the ad hoc holes proximal and distal to the fracture, the plate to the bone before screw insertion. It is critical at this stage to make a thorough assessment of the limb alignment and to establish that the correct rotation has been achieved by comparison with the other limb. Because locking screws are used, the plate cannot be used to effect fracture reduction, which should therefore be achieved before the plate is applied. Additional screws are then inserted percutaneously as necessary, with a minimal of two bicortical screws at either end. Borg and colleagues[32] reported the number of screws that can be placed in a short distal fragment as a limitation of the conventional low-contact plate. This problem has been circumvented by using the ad hoc LP distal tibial plate with nine distal holes instead of the four holes of

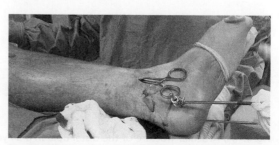

Fig. 2. Through the small incision, the subcutaneous tunnel is created using artery forceps.

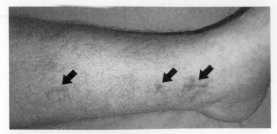

Fig. 3. Final scars (*arrows*) show the minimal nature of the exposure.

the conventional low-contact plate. The latter feature allows modulation of the rigidity of fixation more precisely. Stoffel and colleagues[26] reported the factors that influence stability in compression and torsion. Axial stiffness and torsional rigidity were mainly influenced by the working length (eg, the distance of the first screw to the fracture site). By omitting one screw hole on either side of

the fracture, the construct became almost twice as flexible in compression and torsion. The number of screws also significantly affected stability. More than three screws per fragment did little to increase axial stiffness, however, and four screws did not increase torsional rigidity. The position of the third screw significantly affected axial stiffness but not torsional rigidity. The other factor affecting the stability of the construct is the distance between the plate and the bone, which should be kept small, and long plates should be used to provide sufficient axial stiffness. The optimal plate distance should be 2 mm or less from the surface of the bone.[28] The stab incisions are closed in a standard fashion, the wound is dressed, and the limb is immobilized in a below-the-knee synthetic cast (**Fig. 3**).

Patients are allowed non–weight-bearing crutch walking immediately after surgery. At 2 weeks, the below-the-knee synthetic cast is changed to another short-leg lightweight cast after inspection

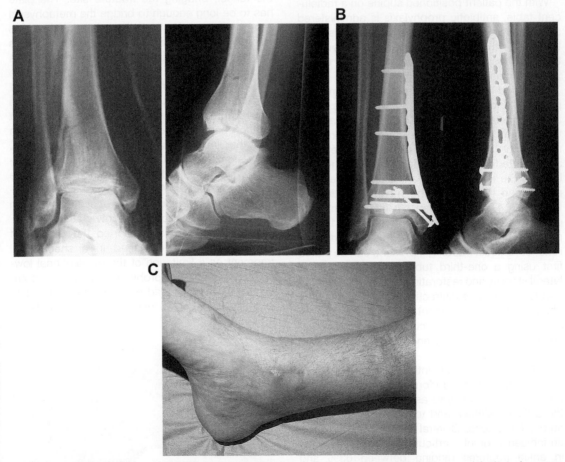

Fig. 4. (*A*) Articular fracture of the distal tibia in a 34-year-old man. (*B*) Six-month follow-up. (*C*) Clinical appearance after 6 months. The patient is fully weight bearing with no walking aids and no limp. Note the well-healed barely visible scars.

of the wound and removal of the sutures. The weight-bearing status depends on the individual fracture pattern, but most patients bear weight at least partially at 6 weeks. Outpatient physiotherapy is instituted to maximize the range of motion of the foot and ankle (**Fig. 4**).

SUMMARY

The management of distal tibia fractures can be challenging because of the scarcity of soft tissue, their subcutaneous nature, and poor vascularity. The timing of surgery should be optimized to allow the soft tissues to stabilize and to minimize the severe postoperative wound problems often associated with the surgical management of these complex fractures. LPs have the biomechanical properties of internal and external fixators, with superior holding power because of fixed angular stability through the head of locking screws, independent of friction fit. Minimally invasive plating techniques reduce iatrogenic soft tissue injury and damage to bone vascularity, in addition to preserving the osteogenic fracture hematoma. Fracture reduction may be more difficult than with open methods. As a consequence of this, the surgeon depends on intraoperative fluoroscopy to confirm that an adequate reduction has been achieved before siting the LP. In periarticular fractures, additional incisions may be needed to visualize and assess the joint surface to ensure that the articular surfaces are anatomically aligned. The cost of the LPs, the technically demanding procedure, and the increased exposure to radiation required to perform the procedure have to be considered when comparing the efficacy of this device with that of normal plates.

REFERENCES

1. Bedi A, Le TT, Karunakar MA. Surgical treatment of nonarticular distal tibia fractures. J Am Acad Orthop Surg 2006;14(7):406–16.
2. Fisher WD, Hamblen DL. Problems and pitfalls of compression fixation of long bone fractures: a review of results and complications. Injury 1978;10(2):99–107.
3. Olerud S, Karlstrom G. Tibial fractures treated by AO compression osteosynthesis. Experiences from a five year material. Acta Orthop Scand Suppl 1972;140:1–104.
4. Francois J, Vandeputte G, Verheyden F, et al. Percutaneous plate fixation of fractures of the distal tibia. Acta Orthop Belg 2004;70(2):148–54.
5. Helfet DL, Shonnard PY, Levine D, et al. Minimally invasive plate osteosynthesis of distal fractures of the tibia. Injury 1997;28(Suppl 1):A42–7 [discussion: A47–8].
6. Maffulli N, Toms AD, McMurtie A, et al. Percutaneous plating of distal tibial fractures. Int Orthop 2004;28(3):159–62.
7. Hasenboehler E, Rikli D, Babst R. Locking compression plate with minimally invasive plate osteosynthesis in diaphyseal and distal tibial fracture: a retrospective study of 32 patients. Injury 2007;38(3):365–70.
8. Hazarika S, Chakravarthy J, Cooper J. Minimally invasive locking plate osteosynthesis for fractures of the distal tibia—results in 20 patients. Injury 2006;37(9):877–87.
9. Lau TW, Leung F, Chan CF, et al. Wound complication of minimally invasive plate osteosynthesis in distal tibia fractures. Int Orthop 2007;16:697–703.
10. Rammelt S, Endres T, Grass R, et al. The role of external fixation in acute ankle trauma. Foot Ankle Clin 2004;9(3):455–74, vii–viii.
11. Boenisch UW, de Boer PG, Journeaux SF. Unreamed intramedullary tibial nailing—fatigue of locking bolts. Injury 1996;27(4):265–70.
12. Vallier HA, Le TT, Bedi A. Radiographic and clinical comparisons of distal tibia shaft fractures (4 to 11 cm proximal to the plafond): plating versus intramedullary nailing. J Orthop Trauma 2008;22(5):307–11.
13. Zelle BA, Bhandari M, Espiritu M, et al. Treatment of distal tibia fractures without articular involvement: a systematic review of 1125 fractures. J Orthop Trauma 2006;20(1):76–9.
14. Im GI, Tae SK. Distal metaphyseal fractures of tibia: a prospective randomized trial of closed reduction and intramedullary nail versus open reduction and plate and screws fixation. J Trauma 2005;59(5):1219–23 [discussion: 1223].
15. Janssen KW, Biert J, van Kampen A. Treatment of distal tibial fractures: plate versus nail: a retrospective outcome analysis of matched pairs of patients. Int Orthop 2007;31(5):709–14.
16. Yang SW, Tzeng HM, Chou YJ, et al. Treatment of distal tibial metaphyseal fractures: plating versus shortened intramedullary nailing. Injury 2006;37(6):531–5.
17. Collinge C, Sanders R, DiPasquale T. Treatment of complex tibial periarticular fractures using percutaneous techniques. Clin Orthop Relat Res 2000;375:69–77.
18. Redfern DJ, Syed SU, Davies SJ. Fractures of the distal tibia: minimally invasive plate osteosynthesis. Injury 2004;35(6):615–20.
19. Cantu RV, Koval KJ. The use of locking plates in fracture care. J Am Acad Orthop Surg 2006;14(3):183–90.
20. Frigg R. Locking compression plate (LCP). An osteosynthesis plate based on the dynamic compression plate and the point contact fixator (PC-Fix). Injury 2001;32(Suppl 2):63–6.
21. Frigg R. Development of the locking compression plate. Injury 2003;34(Suppl 2):B6–10.

22. Wagner M. General principles for the clinical use of the LCP. Injury 2003;34(Suppl 2):B31–42.

23. Carter DR, Beaupre GS, Giori NJ, et al. Mechanobiology of skeletal regeneration. Clin Orthop Relat Res 1998;355(Suppl):S41–55.

24. Greiwe RM, Archdeacon MT. Locking plate technology: current concepts. J Knee Surg 2007;20(1):50–5.

25. Hente R, Fuchtmeier B, Schlegel U, et al. The influence of cyclic compression and distraction on the healing of experimental tibial fractures. J Orthop Res 2004;22(4):709–15.

26. Stoffel K, Dieter U, Stachowiak G, et al. Biomechanical testing of the LCP—how can stability in locked internal fixators be controlled? Injury 2003;34(Suppl 2):B11–9.

27. Tull F, Borrelli J Jr. Soft-tissue injury associated with closed fractures: evaluation and management. J Am Acad Orthop Surg 2003;11(6):431–8.

28. Ahmad M, Nanda R, Bajwa AS, et al. Biomechanical testing of the locking compression plate: when does the distance between bone and implant significantly reduce construct stability? Injury 2007;38(3):358–64.

29. Hintermann B, Regazzoni P, Lampert C, et al. Arthroscopic findings in acute fractures of the ankle. J Bone Joint Surg Br 2000;82(3):345–51.

30. Imade S, Takao M, Nishi H, et al. Arthroscopy-assisted reduction and percutaneous fixation for triplane fracture of the distal tibia. Arthroscopy 2004; 20(10):e123–8.

31. Loren GJ, Ferkel RD. Arthroscopic assessment of occult intra-articular injury in acute ankle fractures. Arthroscopy 2002;18(4):412–21.

32. Borg T, Larsson S, Lindsjo U. Percutaneous plating of distal tibial fractures. Preliminary results in 21 patients. Injury 2004;35(6):608–14.

Percutaneous Hallux Valgus Surgery: A Prospective Multicenter Study of 189 Cases

Thomas Bauer, MD[a,b,*], Christophe de Lavigne, MD[a],
David Biau, MD[a,b], Mariano De Prado, MD[a,c],
Stephen Isham, MD[a,d], Olivier Laffenêtre, MD[a,e]

KEYWORDS

- Hallux valgus • Percutaneous surgery
- Minimally invasive surgery • Metatarsal osteotomy

Hallux valgus is a frequent deformity of the first ray of the foot with progressive abduction and pronation of the first phalanx; adduction, pronation, and elevatus of the first metatarsal, and lateral capsular retraction of the first metatarsophalangeal (MTP) joint.[1–3] Surgical correction of this deformity is classically indicated for painful hallux valgus with shoewear difficulties. Every year, over 200,000 hallux valgus surgical procedures are performed in the United States.[4] Many osteotomies of the first metatarsal have been proposed for the correction of hallux valgus.[3,5–9]

Distal first metatarsal osteotomies have been indicated for the correction of mild-to-moderate deformity with an intermetatarsal angle up to 20° and for the correction of the distal metatarsal articular angle (DMAA).[10,11] Different distal metatarsal osteotomies performed using a minimally invasive percutaneous approach with or without fixation have been proposed.[11–14] The Reverdin osteotomy modified by S. Isham ("Reverdin–Isham" osteotomy) is a minimally invasive procedure allowing an alignment of the first ray by a medial rotation of the head of the first metatarsal and a correction of the DMAA.[12] Using this procedure,

all the osteotomies—bone resection, capsular release, and angular correction—are performed percutaneously with specific instruments, fluoroscopic control, and no fixation. Basically, the percutaneous procedures reduce the surgical trauma and the operating time with potentially fewer complications and quicker recovery. However, with the theoretical drawbacks of stiffness of the first MTP joint and loss of correction, there was speculation about the real benefits of this percutaneous procedure in terms of function and patient satisfaction.[15]

The aim of this study was to assess the results of this percutaneous procedure for the treatment of mild-to-moderate hallux valgus deformity after a minimum 1-year follow-up with regard to functional results, first MTP joint stiffness, patient satisfaction, and correction of the deformities analyzed on radiographs.

SUBJECTS AND METHODS
Study Design

Five departments of orthopaedic surgery participated in this prospective multicenter study. All of

[a] GRECMIP: Groupe de Recherche en Chirurgie Mini-Invasive du Pied, Sport Medical Center, Department of Orthopedic Surgery, 9 rue Jean Moulin, 33700 Merignac, France
[b] Ambroise Paré Hospital, West Paris University, Department of Orthopedic Surgery, 9 Avenue Charles de Gaulle, 92100 Boulogne, France
[c] Hospital San Carlos, 30011 Murcia, Spain
[d] Foot and Ankle Surgery Center, Coeur d'Alene, ID, USA
[e] Bordeaux University Hospital, Department of Orthopedic Surgery, Bordeaux, France
* Corresponding author. Ambroise Paré Hospital, West Paris University, Department of Orthopedic Surgery, 9 Avenue Charles de Gaulle, 92100 Boulogne, France.
E-mail address: thomas.bauer@apr.aphp.fr (T. Bauer).

Orthop Clin N Am 40 (2009) 505–514
doi:10.1016/j.ocl.2009.05.002
0030-5898/09/$ – see front matter © 2009 Elsevier Inc. All rights reserved.

orthopedic.theclinics.com

the subjects who had not undergone prior surgery for hallux valgus and who were undergoing a percutaneous procedure for correction of the deformity between September 2005 and February 2006 were included in the study. The indication for percutaneous surgical procedure was a painful hallux valgus with a mild-to-moderate deformity (hallux valgus angle up to 40° and first intermetatarsal angle up to 15°). Some subjects who had hallux valgus angle greater than 40° but with first intermetatarsal angle less than 15° were included. Other subjects who had hallux valgus angle less than 40° but with first intermetatarsal angle greater than 15° were also included. Subjects who had asymptomatic hallux valgus, severe hallux valgus deformity (hallux valgus angle >40° and intermetatarsal angle >15°), or who had compromised local and systemic conditions (eg, sepsis, neuropathy, severe arteritis), making them poor surgical candidates, were excluded. One hundred eighty-nine feet in 168 consecutive subjects were included in the present study. There were 164 women (185 feet) and four men (4 feet). The median age at time of surgery was 55 years (interquartile range [IQR]: 44–63). There were 97 right feet and 92 left. The subjects were reviewed after surgery within a minimum of 1 year (median follow-up: 13 mo, range: 12 to 24 mo). Ten subjects were excluded from the final results because they missed the follow-up examination, and so the present analysis was performed on 179 feet (Table 1).

Surgical Procedure

All of the procedures were performed under locoregional anesthesia with either popliteal block, ankle block, or distal perimetatarsal block, depending on the preferences of the different surgical teams.

The surgical procedure is based on the description of Isham[12] and De Prado and colleagues.[16] Briefly, the subject was placed in a supine position without tourniquet. Through a 3- to 5-mm incision on the medial plantar aspect of the first metatarsal head, just proximal to the medial sesamoid, the medial capsule of the first MTP joint was gently peeled off of the metatarsal head, and a working area around the medial aspect of the metatarsal head was thus produced. The medial eminence was then resected using a wedge burr with a high-torque, low-speed drill (2000 to 6000 rpm) to avoid bone or skin burn and necrosis (Fig. 1). The extent of bone removal was controlled under fluoroscopy, and bone was removed up to the functional area of the first metatarsal head, medial to the sagittal groove. All of the bony fragments were extruded by pressure on the metatarsal

Table 1 Results of the series			
Data		Preoperative (n = 189)	Postoperative (n = 179)
AOFAS score	Global AOFAS	52 (44–60)	93 (82.5–100)
	Pain	20 (20–20)	40 (30–40)
	Function	29 (24–37)	45 (40–45)
	Alignment	0 (0–0)	15 (15–15)
First MTP joint motion	Range of motion	90° (50–100)	75° (45–100)
	Dorsiflexion	70° (40–80)	60° (35–80)
	Plantar flexion	20° (15–20)	15° (10–20)
Forefoot morphotype	Greek	47 (25%)	48 (27%)
	Square	62 (33%)	88 (49%)
	Egyptian	80 (42%)	43 (24%)
Angles	HV	28° (22–32)	14° (10–18)
	IM	13° (11–15)	10° (9–12)
	DMAA	15° (11–19)	8° (4–10)
Metatarsal index	M1<M2	127 (67%)	125 (70%)
	M1=M2	43 (23%)	45 (25%)
	M1>M2	19 (10%)	9 (5%)
Not congruous MTP joint		28 (15%)	18 (10%)

Clinical and radiological preoperative and postoperative data. For quantitative variables, the median and interquartile range are reported.

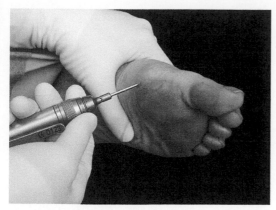

Fig. 1. Bone removal with the wedge burr through the medial plantar portal.

head working area after injection of normosaline into the joint, using rasps to clean the capsule. The Reverdin–Isham osteotomy of the first metatarsal was then performed with a straight burr (**Fig. 2**). This angular medial wedge osteotomy was performed in the distal metaphysis of the first metatarsal, parallel to the joint line from dorsal distal, immediately proximal to the superior articular surface, to plantar proximal, proximal to the sesamoids with a 45° inclination. Care was taken to preserve the lateral cortex. The hallux was then rotated into adductus, and the osteotomy was compressed and closed, correcting at the same time the DMAA (**Fig. 3**). A percutaneous release of the lateral aspect of the MTP joint and abductor tenotomy were then performed with a beaver blade through a lateral dorsal approach over the first MTP joint. A percutaneous Akin

osteotomy of the proximal phalanx of the hallux was then performed through a third 3-mm medial incision, just medial to the tendon of extensor hallucis longus. With a straight burr and under fluoroscopic control, the proximal phalanx of the hallux was osteotomized, preserving the lateral cortex. The medial wedge was then closed by applying a varus stress to the hallux (**Fig. 4**). The osteotomies were stable without internal fixation, and the correction of the deformities was maintained with a crepe bandage. Immediate full weight bearing was allowed with a rigid, flat-soled postoperative shoe for 1 month and no deep venous thrombosis prophylaxis was routinely used. The dressing was removed after the first week, and a cohesive bandage was replaced with an orthoplastic device maintaining first ray alignment (**Fig. 5**). Subjects were encouraged to mobilize the first MTP joint as able after the first week.

Outcome Measures

Clinical assessment
Preoperatively, all subjects underwent an assessment of pain level and functional limitation with use of the American Orthopaedic Foot and Ankle Society's (AOFAS) hallux-metatarsophalangeal-interphalangeal scale (**Table 2**).[17] Additionally, for each subject, passive range of motion of the first MTP joint (the sum of dorsiflexion and plantar flexion) was measured with standard clinical hand-held goniometers with the subject supine, knee flexed at 90° and ankle in neutral position. The digital formula (Greek, square, or Egyptian foot), and hallux valgus deformity reducibility (complete, partial, or no reducibility) were also recorded. Intraoperative data, including associated procedures (eg, extensor hallucis longus percutaneous lengthening, lateral metatarsals percutaneous osteotomies) or intraoperative complications, were accurately noted. Postoperatively, after a minimum 1-year follow-up, all of the subjects included in the present series underwent a new physical examination and assessment with the same data used for the preoperative analysis. The subject's satisfaction with the outcome (very satisfied, satisfied, dissatisfied, or disappointed) was also recorded.

Radiographic assessment
Anteroposterior weight-bearing radiographs were taken preoperatively and at the minimum 1-year follow-up for all subjects. The following measurements were made: the hallux valgus (HV) angle, the first intermetatarsal (IM) angle, the DMAA, and the metatarsal index (M1>M2, M1=M2, M1<M2) were measured. All the measurements were made once manually on actual radiographs

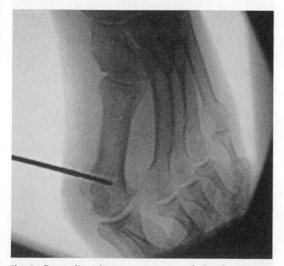

Fig. 2. Reverdin–Isham osteotomy of the first metatarsal with the straight burr.

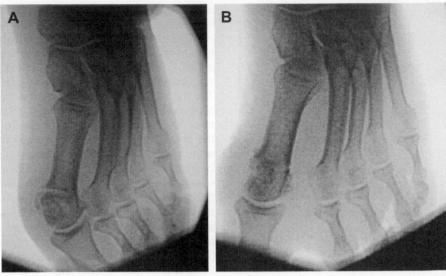

Fig. 3. (*A*) Reverdin–Isham osteotomy before DMAA correction. (*B*) Correction of the DMAA by medial rotation of the first metatarsal head.

by the different investigators participating in this series. The joint congruency of the first MTP was assessed using the criteria defined by Pigott.[2] Arthritis of the MTP joint was evaluated in accordance with the description of Regnauld.[18] The measurements were performed by the different investigators participating in this series (**Fig. 6**).

Statistical analysis

All pre-, intra-, and postoperative data were collected at each participating center by the investigators. For quantitative variables (continuous variables), the median and IQR are reported, unless otherwise specified. Categorical variables are reported as counts. A multivariate analysis with a backward stepwise variable selection procedure, based on Akaike's information criterion,[19] was used to identify a set of independent predictors on the final correction of the deformity (HV angle, IM angle, DMAA), the postoperative dorsiflexion of the first MTP joint and the postoperative congruency of the first MTP joint. The following variables were first tested in univariate models, and only the ones exerting significant influence were entered in the multivariate models: preoperative IM and HV angles, DMAA, associated percutaneous procedures on the lateral rays (yes versus no), percutaneous lengthening of the tendon of extensor hallucis longus (yes versus no), and the presence of osteoarthritis of the first MTP joint on plain radiographs (assessed by the presence or lack of a joint space narrowing). Analyses were adjusted for center effect. All analyses were performed with R 2.5.0 software package.[20]

All tests were two-sided, with a significance level set at $P = .05$.

RESULTS

After a minimum 1-year follow-up, the AOFAS score improved from a preoperative median of 52 points (IQR: 44–60) to a median of 93 points (82.5–100) (see **Table 1**). When dividing the overall AOFAS score into pain, function, and alignment, we observed an improvement from a median

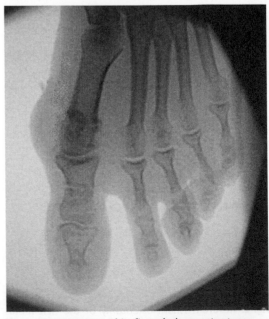

Fig. 4. Percutaneous Akin first phalanx osteotomy.

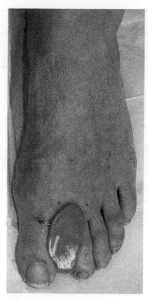

Fig. 5. Postoperative orthoplastic device (1 week postoperative).

preoperative score of 20 points (IQR: 20–20) to 40 points postoperatively (IQR: 30–40) for pain; from a median preoperative score of 29 points (IQR: 24–37) to 45 points postoperatively (IQR: 40–45) for function; and from a median preoperative score of 0 points (IQR: 0-0) to 15 points postoperatively (IQR: 15–15) for alignment. Eighty-seven percent of the subjects (n = 156) were satisfied or very satisfied with the outcome of the procedure at the final follow-up.

The median range of motion of the first MTP joint was 90° (IQR: 55–100) preoperatively (with a median 70° of dorsiflexion [IQR: 40–80] and 20° of plantar flexion [IQR: 15–20]) and 75° (IQR: 45–100) at 1-year follow-up (with a median 60° of dorsiflexion [IQR: 35–80] and 15° of plantar flexion [IQR: 10–20]). Subjects averaged a 17% loss of first MTP joint motion. Multivariate analysis identified only the preoperative first MTP joint range of motion ($P<10^{-4}$; estimate = 0.64; 95% CI = 0.48 to 0.81) and the presence of osteoarthritis of the first MTP joint on plain radiographs (P = .02) as independent predictors of the postoperative range of motion of the first MTP joint.

Radiographic assessment showed an improvement of the median HV angle from 28° (IQR: 22–32) preoperatively to 14° postoperatively (IQR: 10–18). The preoperative HV angle was the only independent predictor of the postoperative HV angle (estimate = 0.29; 95% CI= 0.18 to 0.41; $P<10^{-4}$). The correction of the first MTP valgus deformity averaged 50% of the preoperative deformity. The median first IM angle improved from 13° preoperatively (IQR: 11–15) to 10°

postoperatively (IQR: 9–12). Multivariate analysis identified only the preoperative first IM angle as the predictive factor for the postoperative first IM angle, with a decrease of 20% of the preoperative value (estimate = 0.43; 95% CI= 0.29 to 0.56; $P<10^{-9}$). The median DMAA decreased from 15° preoperatively (IQR: 11–37) to 8° postoperatively (IQR: 4–10), with 37° between the extremes preoperatively and 49° postoperatively.

The following complications were recorded: five subjects developed complex regional pain syndrome (type II), three subjects developed a deep venous thrombosis, and two subjects experienced severe postoperative first MTP joint stiffness necessitating arthrolysis.

DISCUSSION

With a median postoperative AOFAS score of 93 points, the clinical results obtained with this percutaneous procedure for the correction of mild-to-moderate hallux valgus deformity are comparable to those obtained with other percutaneous distal metatarsal osteotomies and to most series of open surgical procedures using chevron, scarf, or proximal metatarsal osteotomies.[6,11,12,14,21–33] Comparing clinical results after hallux valgus surgical correction between series may be difficult because of subject selection and variability of severity of preoperative deformity. However, Freslon and colleagues[34] and Thordarson and colleagues[35] showed that the severity of the preoperative deformity did not correlate with the functional outcome score. Pain relief and improvements in footwear and walking ability are the main expectations for patients before hallux valgus surgery.[36–39] With a significant improvement of the functional score for the different clinical data (pain, function, and alignment) obtained in our subjects after a minimum of one year, the Reverdin-Isham percutaneous procedure seems to be very effective for the functional result of the subjects. Isham[12] reported that 90% of his subjects had an excellent outcome with this procedure, comparable with the 87% of subjects who were satisfied or very satisfied in the present series. The percutaneous procedure presented in this series is at least as effective as traditional procedures for functional results and patient satisfaction.[10–13,22,23,27,32–34,40–47]

Stiffness of the first MTP joint is one of the most feared outcomes after hallux valgus surgery.[10,11,30,32,34,40,46,48,49] By the limited scar on the medial side of the first MTP joint and with extra-articular metatarsal osteotomy, percutaneous procedures theoretically limit the risk of stiffness.[6,11,47] However, the percutaneous

Table 2
American Orthopaedic Foot and Ankle Society's hallux-metatarsaophalangeal-interphalangeal scale[24]

Criteria			Score (Points)
Pain	none		40
	mild, occasional		30
	moderate		20
	severe, constant		0
Functional capability	Activity limitation	none	10
		no limitation of daily activity, limitation of recreational activity	7
		limitation of daily and recreational activity	4
		severe limitation of all activity	0
	Footwear	normal	10
		comfortable and/or insole	5
		orthopaedic	0
	MTP joint motion	>75°	10
		30°–74°	5
		<30°	0
	interphalangeal joint motion	normal	5
		<10°	0
	Joint stability	stable	5
		unstable	0
	Callus	none or asymptomatic	5
		symptomatic	0
Hallux alignment	excellent/good		15
	mild asymptomatic misalignment		8
	symptomatic misalignment		0

From Kitaoka HB, Alexander IJ, Adelaar RS, et al. Clinical rating systems for the ankle—hindfoot, midfoot, hallux and lesser toes. Foot Ankle Int 1994;15:349–53; with permission. Copyright © 2009 by the American Orthopaedic Foot and Ankle Society, Inc.

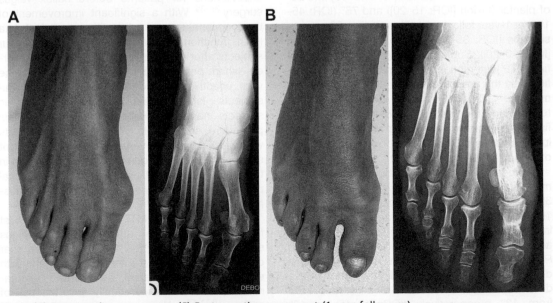

Fig. 6. (*A*) Preoperative assessment. (*B*) Postoperative assessment (1-year follow-up).

procedure performed in this series presents some characteristics that can potentially limit the postoperative MTP joint motion. The extensive bunionectomy produces many bony fragments in the joint and capsular tissues, and is potentially a major cause of joint stiffness. If the working area and the joint are not accurately cleaned with rasps and irrigated with normosaline, the remaining bony fragments may induce an inflammatory reaction leading to pain, fibrosis, and stiffness. Secondly, this modified Reverdin first metatarsal osteotomy is an intracapsular procedure with an increased risk of joint stiffness compared with other percutaneous extra-articular osteotomies.[12,13] With a median loss of $15°$ of the first MTP joint range of motion (corresponding to 17% of the preoperative range of motion), the postoperative stiffness with this procedure is comparable to the stiffness obtained with other percutaneous or open techniques.[30,32,49] In our series, preoperative joint motion was the main predictive factor for postoperative motion. Furthermore, as previously reported, when degenerative joint disease of the first MTP joint was present, subjects had a statistically significant $10°$ loss of dorsiflexion compared with subjects who did not have osteoarthritis.[30]

This percutaneous procedure is effective for the correction of a mild-to-moderate hallux valgus deformity, obtaining an average decrease of 50% of the preoperative first MTP angle (from a mean $28°$ preoperatively to a mean $14°$ postoperatively) and 20% of the preoperative IM angle (from a median $13°$ preoperatively to a median $10°$ postoperatively). These angular corrections are comparable with the reported radiographic results obtained with other percutaneous or open distal metatarsal osteotomies[6,11,13,14,30–32,50,51] or scarf osteotomies.[21,24,25,28,34,41,49,52] There are yet large variations of first MTP angle correction among series of open metatarsal osteotomies (chevron, scarf, or proximal), with investigators reporting a decrease of the deformity larger than 50%[23,25,31,33,47,50,53] and other obtaining only few degrees of correction.[22,23,45,54] Magnan and colleagues[11,14] obtained a greater correction of the IM angle (from $12.3°$ preoperatively to $7.3°$ after a mean follow-up of 3 years with a percutaneous distal metatarsal osteotomy and lateral translation of the first metatarsal head. Maffulli and colleagues[13] obtained a significant reduction of the IM angle (from $11.5°$ preoperatively to $7.5°$ postoperatively) with a minimally invasive distal metatarsal osteotomy similar to the technique described by Magnan and colleagues[11,14] Obviously, for large preoperative metatarsus varus or for greater correction of the IM angle, other metatarsal osteotomies are indicated (chevron, scarf, proximal, or double osteotomy).[23,25,28,30,31,33,34,41,49,51,53]

One of the goals of the modified Reverdin–Isham first metatarsal osteotomy is to decrease the DMAA. In our experience, the mean decrease of the DMAA was 50% (from $15°$ preoperatively to $7°$ at final follow-up). A comparable correction of the DMAA was reported with percutaneous distal metatarsal osteotomy by Magnan and colleagues[11,14] and with chevron osteotomy by Chou and colleagues.[22] Coughlin and Carlson[23] obtained a greater correction of the DMAA (from $23°$ to $9°$) with a double metatarsal osteotomy. Because the possibilities of medial rotation of the plantar metatarsal fragment are limited, the scarf osteotomy allows only few degrees of correction of the DMAA.[25,34,41,52,53] In our series, there are yet large variations in the values of the DMAA, with $37°$ between the extremes preoperatively and $49°$ postoperatively. These findings are first the result of the lack of accuracy and poor reproducibility in the measurement of this angle.[40,55–57] Second, the large variations of the postoperative DMAA confirm that this percutaneous procedure cannot be relied on to give consistent reduction of the DMAA.[47] This lack of accuracy in the adjustment of the first metatarsal head rotation can lead to DMAA undercorrection or increase with a risk of early hallux valgus recurrence or to DMAA overcorrection with a risk of postoperative noncongruency of the first MTP joint. Thus, this percutaneous Reverdin–Isham osteotomy must be indicated only for mild-to-moderate hallux valgus deformity with an increased DMAA.

Unlike Kadakia and colleagues,[15] who report an unacceptably high rate of early complications with percutaneous distal first metatarsal osteotomy, no nonunion, osteonecrosis, or recurrence of hallux valgus deformity were found in our series.

The authors' present study presents several limitations. First, this descriptive series of percutaneous hallux valgus surgery is a short-term follow-up study, and further assessment is necessary to confirm the good clinical results and the absence of loss of correction with time. Second, clinical and radiographic data measurements were not performed by an independent reviewer, but by each investigator; differences between centers could have produced biases and intra- or interobserver reproducibility of the measurements was not assessed.[7,55,56,58,59] However, all analyses were adjusted for each center to diminish the impact of these differences. Finally, all surgeons who participated to the study had several years' experience in percutaneous hallux valgus surgery, and, as a consequence, the results presented may only apply to centers with extensive experience. Percutaneous hallux valgus surgery requires a learning curve, which is not analyzed in the present study, before being able to produce reliably acceptable results. This learning curve includes both surgical technique for osteotomies and postoperative care with dressings and application of appropriate orthoses.

SUMMARY

Percutaneous correction of mild-to-moderate hallux valgus deformity with the Reverdin–Isham osteotomy of the first metatarsal and Akin osteotomy of the proximal phalanx of the hallux enables us to achieve clinical and radiographic results comparable to other percutaneous or open distal metatarsal osteotomies after 1-year follow-up. Further assessments, with measurements of the stability of the angular corrections with time, are required. The risk of postoperative stiffness of the first MTP joint with this procedure is comparable to open techniques, and it underlines the importance of postoperative care and rehabilitation. This procedure does not allow reliable correction of the DMAA, with risks of undercorrection and recurrence, or of overcorrection and joint incongruency. The lack of accuracy of DMAA correction often results from intra- or postoperative difficulties or complications. Experience in percutaneous surgery and postoperative management is probably the main factor for the improvement of long- term results. The Reverdin–Isham osteotomy could be indicated for mild-to-moderate hallux valgus deformities with an increased DMAA.

Further studies with assessment of the time allowed for walking in normal shoes and return to work are required to ascertain whether percutaneous procedures provide social and individual benefits compared with conventional procedures for hallux valgus correction.

REFERENCES

1. Mann RA, Coughlin MJ. Hallux valgus: etiology, anatomy, treatment and surgical considerations. Clin Orthop Relat Res 1981;157:31–41.
2. Pigott H. The natural history of hallux valgus in adolescent and early adult life. J Bone Joint Surg Am 1960;42:749–60.
3. Reverdin J. De la deviation en dehors du gros orteil (hallux valgus, vulg. « oignon », « bunions », « ballen ») et de son traitement chirurgical [Lateral deviation of the hallux (hallux valgus, bunion) and its surgical treatment]. Trans Internat Med Congress 1881;2:508–12 [in French].
4. Coughlin MJ, Thompson FM. The high price of high fashion footwear. Instr Course Lect 1995;44:371–7.
5. Austin DW, Leventen EO. A new osteotomy for hallux valgus: a horizontally directed "V" displacement osteotomy of the metatarsal head for hallux valgus and primus varus. Clin Orthop 1981;157:25–30.
6. Bösch P, Wanke S, Legenstein R. Hallux valgus correction by the method of Bösch: a new technique with a seven-to-ten-year follow-up. Foot Ankle Clin 2000;5:485–98.
7. Cain TD, Boberg J, Ruch JA, et al. Distal metaphyseal osteotomies in hallux abducto valgus surgery. In: McGlamry ED, Banks AS, Downey MS, editors. Comprehensive textbook of foot surgery. 2nd edition. Baltimore (MD): Williams and Wilkins; 1992. p. 493–503.
8. Hawkins FB, Mitchell CL, Hedrick DW. Correction of hallux valgus by metatarsal osteotomy. J Bone Joint Surg 1945;37:387–94.
9. Johnson KA, Cofield RH, Morrey BF. Chevron osteotomy for hallux valgus. Clin Orthop 1979;142:44–7.
10. Klosok JK, Pring DJ, Jessop JH, et al. Chevron or Wilson metatarsal osteotomy for hallux valgus. A prospective randomised trial. J Bone Joint Surg 1993;75B:825–9.
11. Magnan B, Pezze L, Rossi N, et al. Percutaneous distal metatarsal osteotomy for correction of hallux valgus. J Bone Joint Surg Am 2005;87(6):1191–9.
12. Isham SA. The Reverdin–Isham procedure for the correction of hallux abducto valgus. A distal metatarsal osteotomy procedure. Clin Podiatr Med Surg 1991;8(1):81–94.
13. Maffulli N, Oliva F, Coppola C, et al. Minimally invasive hallux valgus correction: a technical note and a feasibility study. J Surg Orthop Adv 2005;14: 193–8.
14. Magnan B, Bortolazzi R, Samaila E, et al. Percutaneous distal metatarsal osteotomy for correction of hallux valgus. Surgical technique. J Bone Joint Surg Am 2006;88(Suppl 1):135–48.
15. Kadakia AR, Smerek JP, Myerson MS. Radiographic results after percutaneous distal metatarsal osteotomy for correction of hallux valgus deformity. Foot Ankle Int 2007;28:355–60.
16. De Prado M, Ripoll PL, Golano P. Hallux valgus. In: Masson, editor. Cirurgia percutanea del pie. Masson (SA): Barcelona; 2003. p. 57–94 [in Spanish].
17. Kitaoka HB, Alexander IJ, Adelaar RS, et al. Clinical rating systems for the ankle—hindfoot, midfoot, hallux and lesser toes. Foot Ankle Int 1994;15:349–53.
18. Regnauld B. Hallux rigidus. In: Elson R, editor. The foot. Berlin, etc: Springer Verlag, 1986;5: p. 92–103.
19. Akaike H. A new look at the statistical model identification. IEEE Trans Automat Contr 1974;19:716–23.
20. R Development Core Team. R: a language and environment. for statistical computing. R Foundation for Statistical Computing, Vienna, Austria. ISBN 3-900051-07-0.

Available at: http://www.R-project.org. Accessed April, 2006.

21. Aminian A, Kelikian A, Moen T. Scarf osteotomy for hallux valgus deformity: an intermediate follow-up of clinical and radiographic outcomes. Foot Ankle Int 2006;27:883–6.

22. Chou LB, Mann RA, Casillas MM. Biplanar chevron osteotomy. Foot Ankle Int 1998;19:579–84.

23. Coughlin MJ, Carlson RE. Treatment of hallux valgus with an increased distal metatarsal articular angle: evaluation of double and triple first ray osteotomies. Foot Ankle Int 1999;20:762–70.

24. Deenik AR, Pilot P, Brandt SE, et al. Scarf versus chevron osteotomy in hallux valgus: a randomized controlled trial in 96 patients. Foot Ankle Int 2007; 28:537–41.

25. Kristen KH, Berger C, Stelzig S, et al. The scarf osteotomy for the correction of hallux valgus deformities. Foot Ankle Int 2002;23:221–9.

26. Portaluri M. Hallux valgus correction by the method of Bösch: a clinical evaluation. Foot Ankle Clin 2000;5:499–511.

27. Radl R, Leithner A, Zacherl M, et al. The influence of personality traits on the subjective outcome of operative hallux valgus correction. Int Orthop 2004;28(5): 303–6.

28. Sanhudo JA. Correction of moderate to severe hallux valgus deformity by a modified chevron shaft osteotomy. Foot Ankle Int 2006;27:581–5.

29. Sanna P, Ruiu GA. Percutaneous distal osteotomy of the first metatarsal (PDO) for the surgical treatment of hallux valgus. Chir Organi Mov 2005; 90(4):365–9.

30. Schneider W, Aigner N, Pinggera O, et al. Chevron osteotomy in hallux valgus: ten-year results of 112 cases. J Bone Joint Surg Br 2004;86:1016–20.

31. Strienstra JJ, Lee JA, Nakadate DT. Large displacement distal chevron osteotomy for the correction of hallux valgus deformity. J Foot Ankle Surg 2002;41: 213–20.

32. Irnka HJ, Zembsch A, Easley ME, et al. The chevron osteotomy for correction of hallux valgus. Comparison of findings after two and five years of follow-up. J Bone Joint Surg Am 2000;82:1373–8.

33. Veri JP, Pirani SP, Claridge R. Crescentic proximal metatarsal osteotomy for moderate to severe hallux valgus: a mean 12,2 year follow-up study. Foot Ankle Int 2001;22:817–22.

34. Freslon M, Gayet LE, Bouche G, et al. Scarf osteotomy for the treatment of hallux valgus: a review of 123 cases with 4,8 years follow-up. Rev Chir Orthop 2005;91:257–66.

35. Thordarson D, Ebramzadeh E, Moorthy M, et al. Correlation of hallux valgus surgical outcome with AOFAS forefoot score and radiological parameters. Foot Ankle Int 2005;26:122–7.

36. Saro C, Jensen I, Lindgren U, et al. Quality-of-life outcome after hallux valgus surgery. Qual Life Res 2007;16:731–8.

37. Schneider W, Knahr K. Metatarsophalangeal and intermetatarsal angle: different values and interpretation of postoperative results dependent on the technique of measurement. Foot Ankle Int 1998;19: 532–6.

38. Thordarson DB, Rudicel SA, Ebramzadeh E, et al. Outcome study of hallux valgus surgery: an AOFAS multi-center study. Foot Ankle Int 2001;22:956–9.

39. Thordarson DB, Ebramzadeh E, Rudicel SA, et al. Age-adjusted baseline data for women with hallux valgus undergoing corrective surgery. J Bone Joint Surg Am 2005;87:66–75.

40. Capasso G, Testa V, Maffulli N, et al. Molded arthroplasty and transfer of the extensor hallucis brevis tendon. A modification of the Keller–Lelievre operation. Clin Orthop Relat Res 1994;308: 43–9.

41. Crevoisier X, Mouhsine E, Ortolano V, et al. The Scarf osteotomy for the treatment of hallux valgus deformity: a review of 84 cases. Foot Ankle Int 2001;22: 970–6.

42. Jardé O, Trinquier-Lautard JL, Meire P, et al. Treatment of hallux valgus by varus osteotomy of the first phalanx associated with adductor plasty. Rev Chir Orthop 1996;82:541–8.

43. Jardé O, Trinquier-Lautard JL, Gabrion A, et al. Hallux valgus treated by Scarf osteotomy of the first metatarsus and the first phalanx associated with an adductor plasty. Apropos of 50 cases with a 2-year follow up. Rev Chir Orthop 1999;85: 374–80.

44. Laffenêtre O, Cermolacce C, Coillard JY, et al. Mini invasive surgery of hallux valgus. In: Valtin B, Leemrijse T, editors. Cahiers d'enseignement de la SOFCOT: Chirurgie de l'avant-pied. Paris: Elsevier SAS; 2005. p. 96–104 [in French].

45. Plaweski S, Eid A, Faure C, et al. Traitement de l'hallux valgus par l'ostéotomie Scarf. A propos de 120 cas [Treatment of hallux valgus deformity with scarf osteotomy: 120 cases]. Rev Chir Orthop 1998;84(Suppl II):67 [in French].

46. Simmonds FA, Menelaus MB. Hallux valgus in adolescents. J Bone Joint Surg Br 1960;42:761–8.

47. Weinberger BH, Fulp JM, Falstrom P, et al. Retrospective evaluation of percutaneous bunionectomies and distal osteotomies without internal fixation. Clin Podiatr Med Surg 1991;8(1):111–36.

48. Jones CP, Coughlin MJ, Grebing BR, et al. First metatarsophalangeal joint motion after hallux valgus correction: a cadaver study. Foot Ankle Int 2005;26: 614–9.

49. Skotak M, Behounek J. Scarf osteotomy for the treatment of forefoot deformity. Acta Chir Orthop Traumatol Cech 2006;73:18–22.

50. Kuo CH, Huang PJ, Cheng YM, et al. Modified Mitchell osteotomy for hallux valgus. Foot Ankle Int 1998;19:585–9.

51. Teli M, Grassi FA, Montoli C, et al. The Mitchell bunionectomy: a prospective study of 60 consecutive cases utilizing single K-wire fixation. J foot Ankle Surg 2001;40:144–51.

52. Salmeron F, Sales de Gauzy J, Galy C, et al. Scarf osteotomy of hallux valgus in children and adolescents. Rev Chir Orthop 2001;87:706–11.

53. Bonnel F, Canovas F, Poiree G, et al. Evaluation of the Scarf osteotomy in hallux valgus related to distal metatarsal articular angle: a prospective study of 79 operated cases. Rev Chir Orthop 1999;85:381–6.

54. Coetzee JC. Scarf osteotomy for hallux valgus repair: the dark side. Foot Ankle Int 2003;24:29–33.

55. Coughlin MJ, Freund E. The reliability of angular measurements in hallux valgus deformities. Foot Ankle Int 2001;22:368–79.

56. Vittetoe DA, Saltzman CL, Krieg JC, et al. Validity and reliability of the first distal metatarsal articular angle. Foot Ankle 1994;15:541–7.

57. Chi TD, Davitt J, Younger A, et al. Intra- and interobserver reliability of the distal metatarsal articular angle in adult hallux valgus. Foot Ankle Int 2002; 22:722–6.

58. Schneider W, Knahr K. Surgery for hallux valgus. The expectations of patients and surgeons. Int Orthop 2001;25:382–5.

59. Schneider W, Csepan R, Knahr K. Reproducibility of the radiographic metatarsophalangeal angle in hallux valgus surgery. J Bone Joint Surg Am 2003;85:494–9.

Bosch Osteotomy and Scarf Osteotomy for Hallux Valgus Correction

Nicola Maffulli, MD, MS, PhD, FRCS (Orth)[a],*,
Umile Giuseppe Longo, MD[b], Francesco Oliva, MD, PhD[c],
Vincenzo Denaro, MD[b], Cristiano Coppola, MD[d]

KEYWORDS

- Minimally invasive • Hallux valgus • Percutaneous
- Bosch • Scarf • Osteotomy

Surgical correction of hallux valgus rebalances the first ray, correcting the various features of the deformity.[1] More than 130 different operative methods have been described for correction of hallux valgus,[1] but the choice of suitable operation remains controversial.[2,3] Distal metatarsal osteotomies have classically been indicated in patients with mild or moderate deformity with an intermetatarsal angle up to 15°,[4] and some distal osteotomies allow the correction of intermetatarsal angles of up to 20°.[5] Distal osteotomies may also be used to correct deformities with deviation of the distal metatarsal articular angle (DMAA) or to address concomitant stiffness. Some studies compared radiographic and clinical results among many different techniques, and satisfaction with most operations is up to 80%.[1,6] In 2004, a systematic review of the published literature concluded that there was no compelling evidence of advantages of any of these methods over any other particular type of surgery.[2]

The scarf osteotomy of the first metatarsal allows strong fixation with early functional recovery[7] and can be combined with other osteotomies and soft tissue procedures.[8] It permits horizontal displacement, shortening, rotation, elevation, and lowering of the metatarsal head.[7,8] The technique can be technically demanding, because it is not a single osteotomy but involves three different cuts, and each of them must be oriented in the optimal direction and plane to be able to produce the right correction. Complications include troughing of the metatarsal with loss of height, delayed union, rotational malunion, recurrence of deformity, and infections.[9,10]

Minimally invasive procedures reduce surgical trauma because they are performed without large incisions, and injury to the soft tissues is limited.[11] Special instruments[12,13] and, in some percutaneous techniques, fluoroscopy are needed.[14] We described a minimal incision distal metatarsal osteotomy technique, requiring no custom instrumentation.[11] The operation is performed under direct vision and without fluoroscopy. In that preliminary feasibility study, the hallux valgus angle in 15 consecutive female patients (21 hallux valgus corrections) preoperatively averaged 32° and decreased to 14.1° at follow-up. We have continued to use the minimal incision approach in treating mild and moderate hallux valgus deformity.

[a] Centre for Sports and Exercise Medicine, Barts and The London School of Medicine and Dentistry, Mile End Hospital, 275 Bancroft Road, London E1 4DG, England, UK
[b] Department of Orthopaedic and Trauma Surgery, Campus Biomedico University, via Alvaro del Portillo, 200 00128 Rome, Italy
[c] Department of Orthopaedics, Università Torvergata, via Montpellier, 1 00100, Rome, Italy
[d] Department of Orthopaedic Surgery, Ospedale Loreto Mare, via Amerigo Vespucci, 26 80142 Napoli, Italy
* Corresponding author.
E-mail address: n.maffulli@qmul.ac.uk (N. Maffulli).

Orthop Clin N Am 40 (2009) 515–524
doi:10.1016/j.ocl.2009.06.003
0030-5898/09/$ – see front matter © 2009 Elsevier Inc. All rights reserved.

orthopedic.theclinics.com

In the present study, we tested the null hypothesis that in patients who have hallux valgus there is no difference between the scarf technique and minimal incision subcapital osteotomy of the first metatarsal regarding (1) duration of surgery, (2) length of hospital stay, (3) American Orthopaedic Foot and Ankle Society (AOFAS) score, (4) Foot and Ankle Outcome Score (FAOS), (5) postoperative hallux valgus angle, (6) postoperative intermetatarsal angle, and (7) postoperative distal metatarsal articular angle. The primary research question was the duration of surgery.

MATERIALS AND METHODS

We selected 72 patients from among a larger group operated for hallux valgus between July 2003 and December 2006. During that time 44 female patients underwent a minimal incision subcapital osteotomy of the first metatarsal for correction of their hallux valgus by one surgeon (Nicola Maffulli, MD, MS, PhD, FRCS[Orth]). From September 2003 to December 2006, 288 patients underwent a scarf osteotomy performed by several orthopedic surgeons (Cristiano Coppola, MD, Francesco Oliva, MD, Vincenzo Denaro, MD). We included patients in the study if they had a hallux valgus angle (HVA) of 20° to 40°,

a 1–2 intermetatarsal angle (IMA) up to 20°, a DMAA up to 25°, no radiographic evidence of degenerative metatarsophalangeal (MTP) arthritis, and persistent symptoms. Patients were excluded if they had had a previous operation on the affected foot, had severe deformity with the intermetatarsal angle greater than 20°, severe degenerative disease or stiffness of the metatarsophalangeal joint, severe instability of the metatarsocruciform or metatarsophalangeal joint, history of diabetes, peripheral vascular disease, peripheral neuropathy, rheumatoid arthritis, or other inflammatory diseases. We also excluded patients who had bilateral hallux valgus, leaving 36 of the 44 patients with the minimal incision operation. Each of the 36 patients in the subcapital osteotomy group (Group 1) was matched, according to their gender, age (±2 years), and intermetatarsal angle (±3°) to a patient who had his/her hallux valgus corrected with a scarf osteotomy. The evaluation of the patients and match of the hallux valgus patients was performed by a senior orthopedic trainee (UGL) who was not involved in the initial treatment of the patients. An agreement was reached after consultation with a fully trained orthopedic surgeon who had not been involved in the treatment when the orthopedic trainee expressed any doubt. A match according to the above criteria

Table 1
Demographic data of the patients included in this study

Variable	Scarf ($N = 36$)	Bosch ($N = 36$)
Age, y ± SD	51.5 ± 3.1	52.6 ± 3
Age range (y)	21–70	19–70
Indication for surgery		
Pain only	6	7
Pain and shoe fit problems	11	10
Pain and cosmetic disturbance	6	5
Pain, shoe fit problems, and cosmetic disturbance	13	14
Pain when wearing shoes	29	31
Heredity: positive family history	24	19
Body mass index (kg/m²)	26.2	26.8
Duration of symptom (y)	15.3 ± 11.2	12.3 ± 6.2
Anesthesia		
Ankle block	11	2
General	6	31
Spinal	19	3
Complications	6	11
Shoes		
Uses same shoes as before surgery	12	15
Need to use wider shoe than before surgery	3	2
Can use smaller shoes than before surgery	21	19

was possible in 36 patients, all women, with a mean age of 51.5 $\pm$ 13.1 years, (range, 21–70 years) (**Table 1**). We did not perform an a priori power analysis. Our institutional ethics review board approved the study, and all patients gave written informed consent to participate.

We performed preoperative evaluations the day before surgery. Each patient was evaluated for duration and type of preoperative symptoms, pre- and postoperative range of motion (ROM), pre- and postoperative AOFAS[15] clinical rating system for the hallux, and FAOS.[16] The presence of callosities, any deformity of the other toes, and a history of metatarsalgia was also documented.[17] Pain on motion in the first MTP joint (yes or no) also was recorded.

All patients received a standard preoperative assessment using standard radiographs. Standardized anteroposterior and lateral radiographs during weight-bearing were made preoperatively, at 1 year, and at the last postoperative follow-up. The minimum follow-up was 2.1 years (mean, 2.5 years; range, 2.1–3.2 years).

The minimal incision distal osteotomy was also performed under general anesthesia with the patient supine; the foot was prepared in the standard fashion and exsanguinated. A calf tourniquet was used. Soft tissue release was not needed, given the large lateral shift of the metatarsal head achievable. If stiffness of the metatarsophalangeal joint was present, we manually stretched the adductor hallucis, forcing the hallux into a varus position before the skin incision. A 2-cm medial incision was made just proximal to the bunion. The incision was deepened through the skin, subcutaneous tissue, and the medial aspect of the first metatarsal was exposed. We retracted the soft tissues dorsally and plantarward. A 2-mm Kirschner wire was inserted, using a drill passing through the incision into the soft tissue adjacent to the distal end of the first metatarsal and the hallux in a proximal-to-distal direction parallel to the longitudinal axis of the hallux. The Kirschner wire exited just medial to the tip of the hallux close to the nail, and was retracted up to the proximal end. An osteotomy was performed using a standard pneumatic saw with a 9.5 $\times$ 25 $\times$ 0.4-mm blade (Hall Surgical Linvatec Corporation, Largo, Florida). Using different inclinations of the bone cut and different displacements of the head (lateral, dorsal, plantar, medial tilt, or rotation), it is possible to correct each component of the deformity.[18]

With a small osteotome, we mobilized the head of the first metatarsal. We obtained the correction by translating the metatarsal head laterally. The osteotomy was stabilized by inserting a Kirschner

wire into the medullary canal of the first metatarsal in a distal-to-proximal direction to the base of the first metatarsal. After ensuring that no dorsal migration of the head of the first metatarsal had occurred, another 2-mm Kirschner wire was inserted in a proximal-to-distal and medial-to-lateral direction, from the medial and dorsal aspect of the metatarsal shaft, 12 mm proximal to the subcapital osteotomy, directing it toward the head of the first metatarsal to further stabilize the osteotomy. This Kirschner wire was removed 2 weeks after the operation. The skin was sutured, and the protruding Kirschner wires were curved and cut. We did not perform a lateral release with dissection of the lateral soft tissues of the hallux (**Figs. 1–6**).

The scarf osteotomy was performed under general anesthesia with the patient supine; the foot was prepared in the standard fashion and exsanguinated. We used a calf tourniquet. A 6-cm straight medial incision was made to expose the medial aspect of the first metatarsal and metatarsophalangeal joint (MTPJ) capsule. We incised the MTPJ capsule longitudinally to expose the medial eminence and joint. A 2-cm incision was made between the first and second metatarsals to visualize the lateral joint capsule. The lateral MTPJ capsule was incised longitudinally to allow the sesamoids to reduce under the metatarsal head. With the lateral aspect of the first metatarsal exposed, we performed a three-cut Z osteotomy. The distal cut was made 5 mm proximal to the articular surface of the first metatarsal. This cut was made from dorsal to plantar, whereas the proximal cut was made from plantar to dorsal.

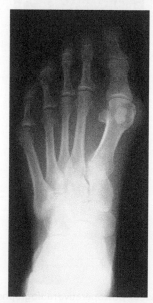

Fig. 1. Preoperative radiographs of a hallux valgus managed with a minimal incision osteotomy.

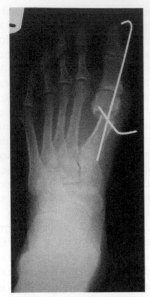

Fig. 2. Postoperative radiographs of a hallux valgus managed with a minimal incision osteotomy.

The proximal cut began approximately 4 cm more proximal in the metatarsal shaft. The longitudinal osteotomy corrected the two other limbs. We then translated the plantar/distal portion laterally to close the intermetatarsal gap and secured the osteotomy with two minifragment screws (2 mm or 2.7 mm in diameter). The exposed medial eminence and dorsomedial metatarsal shaft were removed. The medial joint capsule was repaired and the wound closed. Following the medial

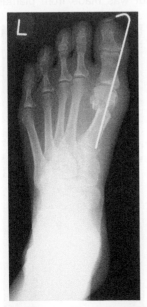

Fig. 3. Two-week postoperative radiographs of a hallux valgus managed with a minimal incision osteotomy, after removal of one Kirschner wire.

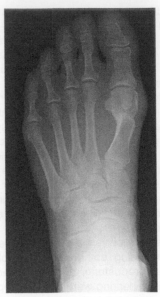

Fig. 4. Two-year postoperative radiographs of a hallux valgus managed with a minimal incision osteotomy.

capsulorrhaphy, to correct any residual hallux valgus interphalangeal or pronation deformity,[8,19,20] we performed an Akin osteotomy of the base of the proximal phalanx of the hallux and fixed the osteotomy with a single minifragment screws (2 mm) or with a metal staple. This osteotomy was performed in 21 of the 36 patients.

In both groups, we applied a bulky compressive bandage after completion of surgery and obtained radiographs (anteroposterior and oblique views). We allowed immediate assisted walking with crutches for 2 weeks recommending that the patient walk on the heel, and foot elevation was

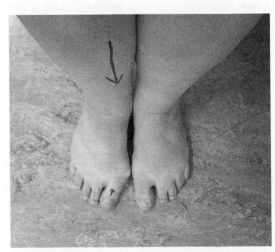

Fig. 5. Preoperative clinical picture of a patient managed with a minimal incision osteotomy.

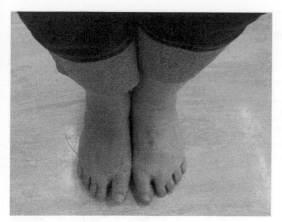

Fig. 6. Postoperative clinical picture of a hallux valgus managed with a minimal incision osteotomy.

advised when at rest. All the operations were planned with at least one overnight stay in hospital, but the decision to discharge the patient was based on the patient's comfort and the ability to negotiate steps with crutches. At 2 weeks, the bandages were completely removed in all patients.

In the patients who had the minimal incision osteotomy, we removed the Kirschner wire inserted in a proximal-to-distal and medial-to-lateral direction, from the medial and dorsal aspect of the metatarsal shaft. The foot was bandaged again with a felt spacer between the hallux and the second toe; we recommended that the patients walk on the heel and advised foot elevation when at rest. After 6 weeks, the dressing and the remaining Kirschner wire were removed.

In the patients who had a scarf osteotomy, the bandage was reduced to a light dressing with a felt spacer between the hallux and the second toe. For patients undergoing a scarf osteotomy, the bulky dressing was removed at 2 weeks, when passive and active mobilization of the metatarsophalangeal and interphalangeal joint was started. The surgical boot was recommended for a further 2 weeks. At that stage, weight-bearing as able with no walking aids was allowed.

Six weeks after the operation, all bandages were removed, and cycling and swimming were encouraged in all patients. Patients were told to wear comfortable normal shoes for 3 to 6 months, gradually returning to former footwear. Patients were advised to use a spacer between the hallux and the second toe for 3 months after the operation at night.

Postoperatively patients were evaluated for AOFAS score and FAOS, and standard radiographs were taken at 2 weeks, 6 weeks, 1 year, and 2 years postoperatively.

Measurements were performed on all patients at a later date in a random order by one trained independent observer (UGL). The HVA was determined by two intersecting lines. The first line was drawn from the center of the first metatarsal head through the center of the base of the first metatarsal.[21] The second line was drawn from the center of the proximal articular surface of the proximal phalanx through the center of the distal end of the diaphysis. This method with reference points distal and proximal to the osteotomy site has good measurement reproducibility. We have previously shown this measure has an average intertester variability of 1.2°, and an average intratester variability of 1.1°.[1,11] To measure the IMA, we used the angle formed by the intersection of the longitudinal axis of the first metatarsal and the second metatarsal (a line drawn through the center of the distal articular surface and the center of the proximal end of the diaphysis). This measurement method has a reported average intertester variability of 1°, and an average intratester variability of 1°. The position of the sesamoids was assigned a grade of 0 to 4.[1,6]

The DMAA was determined as previously described.[22] Six degrees or less was defined as a normal DMAA. From preoperative and postoperative radiographs, the lengths of the first and second metatarsals were measured in millimeters, and the percentage shortening of the first metatarsal was expressed as a/b before operation, divided by a′/b′ at review, multiplied by100, as we previously described.[1] This ratio was used in all linear measurements.

We calculated descriptive statistics. Using the Wilcoxon sign rank test we then compared the following parameters between the groups: (1) duration of surgery, (2) length of hospital stay, (3) AOFAS score at last follow-up, (4) FAOS at last follow-up, (5) postoperative HVA, (6) postoperative IMA, and (7) postoperative DMAA. A post hoc Bonferroni correction was performed, because we performed a total of 14 multiple comparisons.

RESULTS

There were no differences in FAOS and AOFAS scores both pre- and postoperatively comparing the scarf and the minimal incision distal osteotomy (**Tables 2–4**).

The mean operative time for the scarf osteotomy was greater ($P = 0.0024$) that that for the osteotomy (42 minutes with a range of 31–84 minutes versus 19 minutes with a range of 11–29 minutes) (**Table 1**).

In Group 1 (scarf osteotomy), the length of hospital stay was 2.1 ± 1.4 days (range, 1–3

Table 2
American Orthopaedic Foot and Ankle Society clinical rating system scores before surgery and at final follow-up

Osteotomy	Total (100 Points)		Pain (40 Points)		Function (45 Points)		Alignment (15 Points)	
	Pre	Post	Pre	Post	Pre	Post	Pre	Post
Scarf	51 ± 13	86 ± 8	21 ± 10	38 ± 8	28 ± 8	39 ± 10	2 ± 3	15 ± 5
Bosch	54 ± 10	85 ± 11	21 ± 9	39 ± 10	28 ± 10	33 ± 9	2 ± 3	13 ± 5

Mean values $\pm$ SD. Best possible score is indicated within parentheses.

days). In Group 2 (minimal incision distal osteotomy), the length of hospital stay was 1.1 ± 0.4 days (range, 0–2 days) ($P = .041$).

In Group 1 (scarf osteotomy), the AOFAS score increased from 51 ± 13 to 86 ± 8, with 16 patients reporting a fully normal hallux ($P = .036$). In Group 2 (minimal incision distal osteotomy) the AOFAS score increased from 54 ± 10 to 85 ± 11, with 19 patients reporting a fully normal hallux ($P = .033$) **(Table 2)**.

In Group 1 (scarf osteotomy), the overall FAOS improved from a preoperative average rating of 258 ± 22 (range, 178–293) to an average of 358 ± 29 (range, 299–401) postoperatively ($P = .038$). In Group 2 (minimal incision distal osteotomy), the FAOS improved from a preoperative average rating of 264 ± 19 (range, 182–300) to a postoperative average of 356 ± 28 (range, 302–402) ($P = .033$) **(Table 4)**.

In Group 1 (scarf osteotomy), the hallux valgus angle improved from a preoperative average of $28° \pm 6°$ (range, 17°–38°) to an average of $20° \pm 6°$ (range, 9°–22°) postoperatively ($P = .04$). In

Group 2 (minimal incision distal osteotomy) the hallux valgus angle improved from a preoperative average of $27° \pm 6°$ (range, 19°–40°) to an average of $17° \pm 4°$ (range, 8°–22°) postoperatively ($P = .03$). In Group 1 (scarf osteotomy), the intermetatarsal angle improved from a preoperative average rating of $14° \pm 3°$ (range, 10°–18°) to an average of $8° \pm 4°$ (range, 2°–11°) postoperatively ($P = .04$). In Group 2 (minimal incision distal osteotomy), the intermetatarsal angle improved from a preoperative average rating of $15° \pm 6°$ (range, 10°–19°) to an average of $8° \pm 1°$ (range, 1°–3°) postoperatively ($P = .041$). In Group 1 (scarf osteotomy), the average DMAA decreased from $12° \pm 6°$ (range, 5°–20°) preoperatively to $7° \pm 5°$ (range, 4°–11°; $P = .03$). In Group 2 (minimal incision distal osteotomy), the average DMAA decreased from $11° \pm 5°$ (range, 5°–18°) preoperatively to $7° \pm 4°$ (range, 4°–12°; $P = .03$).

Three patients in the minimal incision distal osteotomy group experienced a skin reaction around the Kirschner wire exit at the tip of the hallux. They received oral antibiotics, elevation, and rest with

Table 3
Clinical and radiographic details

	Scarf			Mini-Incision Osteotomy		P Value
Duration of surgery	42 ± 12.4 min (range, 31–84 min)			19 ± 7.3 min (range, 11–29 min)		.0024
Length of hospital stay	2.1 ± 1.4 d (range, 1–3 d)			1.1 ± 0.4 d (range, 0–2 d)		.041
	Preoperative	Postoperative	P value	Preoperative	Postoperative	P value
AOFAS	51 ± 13	86 ± 8	.036	54 ± 10	85 ± 11	.033
FAOS	258 ± 22 (range 178–293)	358 ± 29 (range, 299–401)	.038	264 ± 19 (range, 182–300)	356 ± 28 (range, 302–402)	.033
Hallux valgus angle	28 ± 6	20 ± 6	.04	27 ± 6	17 ± 4	.03
Intermetatarsal angle	14 ± 3	8 ± 4	.04	15 ± 6	8 ± 3	.041
Distal metatarsal articular angle	$12° \pm 6°$	$7° \pm 5°$	.03	$11° \pm 5°$	$7° \pm 4°$	.03

Table 4
Foot and Ankle Outcome Score (FAOS) subscores (mean ± SD) before surgery and at final follow-up on a 0–100 worst–best scale

Osteotomy	Total (500 Points)		Pain (100 Points)		Other Symptoms (100 Points)		Function in Daily Living (100 Points)		Function in Sport and Recreation (100 Points)		Foot and Ankle–Related Quality of Life (100 Points)	
	Pre	Post	Pre	Post	Pre	Post	Pre	Post	Pre	Post	Pre	Post
Scarf	258 ± 22	358 ± 29	57 ± 18	81 ± 16	59 ± 16	75 ± 13	67 ± 18	88 ± 16	41 ± 19	55 ± 22	33 ± 14	59 ± 20
Bosch	264 ± 19	356 ± 28	59 ± 13	83 ± 16	60 ± 8	77 ± 17	69 ± 21	83 ± 21	42 ± 21	53 ± 26	33 ± 15	60 ± 27

Mean values ± SD. Best possible score is indicated within parentheses.

no adverse effect. In a patient who kept the tip of the Kirschner wire uncovered, 4 weeks after the index procedure this became dislodged. The patient received bandaging and a spacer between the hallux and the second toe. The correction obtained at surgery was partially lost, but the patient was satisfied with the cosmetic result. Another patient kept the tip of the Kirschner wire uncovered and 2 weeks after the index procedure presented with a soft tissue infection positive for *Pasteurella multocida*. She reported that her cat had licked her toes on several occasions. The patient was admitted for elevation and amoxicillin and clavulanic acid (625 mg orally three times a day) and ciprofloxacin (500 mg orally twice a day) for 7 days and made an uneventful recovery. The Kirschner wire was kept in situ and was removed, as planned, at 6 weeks from the index procedure. In the two patients who reported discomfort from the sharp edge of the proximal portion of the first metatarsal at the osteotomy site, this was trimmed under local anesthesia 6 months after the index procedure. In the scarf group, the first metatarsal fractured intraoperatively and necessitated fixation with a plate in three patients. The final result was not affected by this inconvenience. Five patients required removal of the screws used for fixation, as they were prominent over the dorsum of the first metatarsal, and caused irritation of the skin when wearing shoes.

DISCUSSION

Minimally invasive distal metatarsal osteotomies have challenged objectives in forefoot surgery, attempting to obtain good clinical results with the least damage to anatomic structures.[23,24] The rationale of our study was to compare the duration of surgery, the length of hospital stay, the AOFAS score, the FAOS score, the hallux valgus angle, and the intermetatarsal angle in patients with hallux valgus surgically managed with scarf or minimal incision distal osteotomy.

There are limitations in the present study. Although ours was a retrospective case control study we did not perform an a priori power analysis. Rather, we limited the number of patients to enroll in the study according to what we knew our unit could deliver within the time we chose to allocate to the study. Our preliminary findings need to be confirmed at longer follow-up and with larger patient populations.

When compared with the scarf osteotomy, the minimal incision distal osteotomy technique produces comparable AOFAS score, FAOS, postoperative HVA, and postoperative IMA, but shorter duration of surgery and length of hospital stay.

Table 5
Comparison of our data with those in the literature for each key variable

Study	Mean Follow-up	AOFAS Preop	AOFAS Postop	FAOS Score Preop	FAOS Score Postop	Duration of Surgery	Length of Hospital Stay	Preop Hallux Valgus Angle	Postop Hallux Valgus Angle	Preop Intermeta Tarsal Angle	Postop Interme Tatarsal Angle	Preop DMAA	Postop DMAA
Barragan-Hervella et al, 2008[25]	6 mo	60.37 (95% CI, 53.87–66.38)	96.62 (95% CI, 94.63–98.70)	Not reported	Not reported	Not reported	Not reported	Not reported	Not reported	Not reported	Not reported	Not reported	Not reported
Bösch et al, 2000[12]	8 y	Not reported	Not reported	Not reported	Not reported	Not reported	Not reported	36 (14–54)	19 (7–4)	13 (6–18)	10 (3–18)	Not reported	Not reported
Portaluri, 2000[13]	16.4 mo (range, 6–27 mo)	Not reported	Not reported	Not reported	Not reported	Not reported	Not reported	27 ± 9 (11–53)	10 ± 7 (0–31)	14 ± 6 (4–26)	7 ± 3 (0–15)	14 ± 6 (2–27)	7 ± 5 (0–18)
Giannini et al, 2003[18]	36 mo (range, 22–52 mo)	Not reported	81	Not reported	Not reported	Not reported	Not reported	Not reported	Not reported	Not reported	Not reported	Not reported	Not reported
Giannini et al, 2007[26]	4 y (range, 2–6 y)	43 (10–75)	88 (52–100)	Not reported	Not reported	Not reported	Not reported	33 (18–60)	16 (2–36)	13 (11–24)	7 (0–16)	Not reported	Not reported
Kadakia et al, 2007[27]	130 d (range, 50–207 d)	Not reported	Not reported	Not reported	Not reported	Not reported	Not reported	25 (16–33)	12 (1–24)	10.3 (7–14)	6.4 (2–10)	Not reported	Not reported
Leemrijse et al, 2008[28]	Not reported	Not reported	Not reported	Not reported	Not reported	Not reported	1.5 d	Not reported	Not reported	Not reported	Not reported	Not reported	Not reported
Magnan et al, 2005[29]	35.9 ± 10.9 mo (range, 24–78 mo)	Not reported	88.2 ± 12.9	Not reported	Not reported	Not reported	Not reported	31.5 ± 10.2 (18–42)	13.7 ± 6.7 (7–25)	12.3 ± 3 (10–20)	7.3 ± 2.7 (4–16)	Not reported	Not reported
Magnan et al, 2006[14]	35.9 ± 10.9 mo (range, 24–78 mo)	Not reported	88.2 ± 12.9	Not reported	Not reported	Not reported	Not reported	31.5 ± 10.2 (18–42)	13.7 ± 6.7 (7–25)	12.3 ± 3 (10–20)	7.3 ± 2.7 (4–16)	Not reported	Not reported
Magnan et al, 2008[30]	35.9 ± 10.9 mo (range, 24–78 mo)	Not reported	88.2 ± 12.9	Not reported	Not reported	Not reported	Not reported	31.5 ± 10.2 (18–42)	13.7 ± 6.7 (7–25)	12.3 ± 3 (10–20)	7.3 ± 2.7 (4–16)	Not reported	Not reported
Maffulli et al, 2005[11]	25 ± 3.2 mo	Not reported	Not reported	Not reported	Not reported	Not reported	Not reported	32 ± 12 (range, 28–42)	14.1 ± 4.7 (range, 7.5–22)	11.5 ± 4 (range, 10–17)	7.5 ± 3 (range, 3–11)	13.1 ± 6.2 (range, 5.5–21.5)	7 ± 4.2 (range, 5–12)
Sanna and Ruiu, 2005[32]	31.5 (range, 25–46 mo)	Not reported	Not reported	Not reported	Not reported	Not reported	Not reported	32 (range 14–55)	12.5	15 (range, 10–23)	9.1	15.6	3
Maffulli et al, present study	2.5 y (range, 2.1–3.2 y)	54 ± 10	85 ± 11	264 ± 19 (range, 182–300)	356 ± 28 (range, 302–402)	19 ± 7.3 min (range, 11–29 min)	1.1 ± 0.4 d (range, 0–2 d)	27 ± 6	17 ± 4	15 ± 6	8 ± 3	11 ± 5	7 ± 4

Only the data that were reported in each study are reported in the table.

This finding may benefit the patients and has financial implications for the hospital. It is difficult to compare the findings of the present study with those of previous reports, because we know of no other studies to compare the clinical outcome of surgical correction of hallux valgus using minimal incision distal osteotomy or scarf technique. Although scarf osteotomy is well established for the management of hallux valgus, no studies focused on the comparison between this technique and minimal incision distal osteotomy. To compare or contrast our data on Bosch osteotomy for hallux valgus correction related to each question of our investigation with those in the literature, we conducted a comprehensive literature search of Medline, EMBASE, Cochrane, CINAHL, and Google Scholar, using the keywords "hallux valgus," "minimally invasive," "percutaneous," "Bosch," "subcutaneous metatarsal first osteotomy (SCOT)," "SERI (simple, effective, rapid, inexpensive)," "PDO (percutaneous distal osteotomy)" over the years 1966 to 2009. All journals were considered, all relevant articles were retrieved, and their bibliographies searched for further references. Given the linguistic capabilities of the research team, we considered publications in English, Italian, French, Spanish, and Portuguese. The search was limited to articles published in peer-reviewed journals. We excluded technical notes, literature reviews, letters to editors, and articles not specifically reporting outcomes. This process left us with a total of 14 articles, all of which dealt with minimal incision correction of the hallux valgus.[11–14,18,25–32] A table is provided (Table 5) to synthesize our data with those in the literature for each key variable of our study.

Giannini and colleagues[18,26] summarized the characteristics of the minimal incision technique of correction of the hallux valgus with the abbreviation SERI (simple, effective, rapid, inexpensive). In their first report,[18] the authors stated that the surgical time spent was approximately 5 minutes, even though no specific data on duration of surgery were presented in an extensive way in the article. In our study, the duration of surgery was less in the minimal incision osteotomy group than in the scarf osteotomy group; this is not surprising, given the exposure required for the scarf osteotomy and the number of steps that such a procedure involves. We caution, however, against choosing one procedure over another based just on the length of the operation.

Leemrijse and colleagues[28] reported that patients who underwent minimally invasive procedures had a mean hospital length of stay of 1.5 days, shorter when compared with patients undergoing conventional procedures for the correction of the hallux valgus,[28] resulting in financial benefit for the hospital.[28] In our setting, we planned that our patients be discharged after at least one overnight stay in hospital, but the decision to discharge the patient was based on the patient's comfort and ability to negotiate steps with crutches. We expected interindividual variability, but it does seem that the less invasive procedure would allow planning for patients to have a short hospital stay. Indeed, as our confidence using this procedure has increased, in patients who necessitate only hallux valgus correction we now undertake the procedure on an outpatient basis.

The results of the AOFAS score, HVA, IMA, and DMAA in our study were comparable to those in the literature of similar reports on minimally invasive surgery for hallux valgus correction (Table 5).

FAOS has not been used in the other retrieved studies, and therefore a strict comparison of our results with the literature is not possible.

Our study confirmed the benefits of a minimal incision distal metatarsal osteotomy. The minimal incision distal osteotomy allows the orthopedic surgeon to reliably correct most hallux valgus deformities without removing the bunion and without open lateral release, performing only a manipulation of the big toe. The clinical and radiographic results are comparable to those obtainable with the scarf osteotomy, but our results are not as clinically and radiographically impressive as those reported by other investigators using a similar technique.[33] The procedure allows shorter operating time and earlier discharge with lower risk for complications due to surgical exposure, including minimal soft tissue dissection, decreased risk for vascular disruption secondary to a lack of capsular disruption, avoidance of lateral cortex penetration with the saw, and high union rate given the minimal soft tissue disruption. It seems intuitive that minimal incision techniques would be beneficial in the high-risk patient who has an ulceration or recurrent ulceration as a means of performing limb preservation/salvage without extensive soft tissue and osseous trauma.[23,24] Additional mechanical and clinical investigations are needed to understand the role of the minimal incision technique in the management of patients with hallux valgus.

REFERENCES

1. Klosok JK, Pring DJ, Jessop JH, et al. Chevron or Wilson metatarsal osteotomy for hallux valgus. A prospective randomised trial. J Bone Joint Surg Br 1993;75(5):825–9.

2. Ferrari J, Higgins JP, Prior TD. Interventions for treating hallux valgus (abductovalgus) and bunions. Cochrane Database Syst Rev 2004;(1):CD000964.

3. Saro C, Andrén B, Wildemyr Z, et al. Outcome after distal metatarsal osteotomy for hallux valgus: a prospective randomized controlled trial of two methods. Foot Ankle Int 2007;28(7):778–87.

4. Chang JT, et al. Distal metaphyseal osteotomies in hallux abducto valgus surgery. In: Banks AS, Downey MS, Martin DE, et al, editors. McGlamry's comprehensive textbook of foot and ankle surgery. Philadelphia: Lippincott; 2001. p. 505–27.

5. Mizuno K, Hashimura M, Kimura M, et al. Treatment of hallux valgus by oblique osteotomy of the first metatarsal. Foot Ankle 1992;13(8):447–52.

6. Capasso G, Testa V, Maffulli N, et al. Molded arthroplasty and transfer of the extensor hallucis brevis tendon. A modification of the Keller-Lelievre operation. Clin Orthop Relat Res 1994;(308):43–9.

7. Weil LS. Scarf osteotomy for correction of hallux valgus. Historical perspective, surgical technique, and results. Foot Ankle Clin 2000;5(3):559–80.

8. Barouk LS. Scarf osteotomy for hallux valgus correction. Local anatomy, surgical technique, and combination with other forefoot procedures. Foot Ankle Clin 2000;5(3):525–58.

9. Sammarco GJ, Idusuyi OB. Complications after surgery of the hallux. Clin Orthop Relat Res 2001;(391):59–71.

10. Lipscombe S, Molloy A, Sirikonda S, et al. Scarf osteotomy for the correction of hallux valgus: midterm clinical outcome. J Foot Ankle Surg 2008;47(4): 273–7.

11. Maffulli N, Oliva F, Coppola C, et al. Minimally invasive hallux valgus correction: a technical note and a feasibility study. J Surg Orthop Adv 2005;14(4):193–8.

12. Bosch P, Wanke S, Legenstein R. Hallux valgus correction by the method of Bosch: a new technique with a seven-to-ten-year follow-up. Foot Ankle Clin 2000;5(3):485–98, v–vi.

13. Portaluri M. Hallux valgus correction by the method of Bosch: a clinical evaluation. Foot Ankle Clin 2000;5(3):499–511, vi.

14. Magnan B, Bortolazzi R, Samaila E, et al. Percutaneous distal metatarsal osteotomy for correction of hallux valgus. Surgical technique. J Bone Joint Surg Am 2006;88(Suppl1 Pt 1):135–48.

15. Kitaoka HB, Alexander IJ, Adelaar RS, et al. Clinical rating systems for the ankle-hindfoot, midfoot, hallux, and lesser toes. Foot Ankle Int 1994;15(7): 349–53.

16. Roos EM, Brandsson S, Karlsson J. Validation of the foot and ankle outcome score for ankle ligament reconstruction. Foot Ankle Int 2001;22(10):788–94.

17. Brooks R. EuroQol: the current state of play. Health Policy 1996;37:53–72.

18. Giannini S, Ceccarelli F, Bevoni R, et al. Hallux valgus surgery: the minimally invasive bunion correction. Tech Foot Ankle Surg 2003;2:11–20.

19. Coughlin MJ, Smith BW. Hallux valgus and first ray mobility. Surgical technique. J Bone Joint Surg Am 2008;90(Suppl2 Pt 2):153–70.

20. Coughlin MJ, Jones CP. Hallux valgus and first ray mobility. A prospective study. J Bone Joint Surg Am 2007;89(9):1887–98.

21. Schneider W, Csepan R, Kasparek M, et al. Intra- and interobserver repeatability of radiographic measurements in hallux surgery: improvement and validation of a method. Acta Orthop Scand 2002; 73(6):670–3.

22. Richardson EG, Graves SC, McClure JT, et al. First metatarsal head-shaft angle: a method of determination. Foot Ankle 1993;14(4):181–5.

23. Roukis TS. Central metatarsal head-neck osteotomies: indications and operative techniques. Clin Podiatr Med Surg 2005;22(2):197–222, vi.

24. Roukis TS, Schade VL. Minimum-incision metatarsal osteotomies. Clin Podiatr Med Surg 2008;25(4): 587–607, viii.

25. Barragan-Hervella RG, Morales-Flores F, Arratia-Rios M, et al. [Clinical results of hallux valgus minimally surgery]. Acta Ortop Mex 2008;22(3):150–6 [in Spanish].

26. Giannini S, Vannini F, Faldini C, et al. The minimally invasive hallux valgus correction (S.E.R.I). Interact Surg 2007;2:17–23.

27. Kadakia AR, Smerek JP, Myerson MS. Radiographic results after percutaneous distal metatarsal osteotomy for correction of hallux valgus deformity. Foot Ankle Int 2007;28:355–60.

28. Leemrijse T, Valtin B, Besse JL. [Hallux valgus surgery in 2005. Conventional, mini-invasive or percutaneous surgery? Uni- or bilateral? Hospitalisation or one-day surgery?]. Rev Chir Orthop Reparatrice Appar Mot 2008;94(2):111–27 [in French].

29. Magnan B, Pezze L, Rossi N, et al. Percutaneous distal metatarsal osteotomy for correction of hallux valgus. J Bone Joint Surg Am 2005;87(6):1191–9.

30. Magnan B, Samaila E, Viola G, et al. Minimally invasive retrocapital osteotomy of the first metatarsal in hallux valgus deformity. Oper Orthop Traumatol 2008;20(1):89–96.

31. Migues A, Campaner G, Slullitel G, et al. Minimally invasive surgery in hallux valgus and digital deformities. Orthopedics 2007;30(7):523–6.

32. Sanna P, Ruiu GA. Percutaneous distal osteotomy of the first metatarsal (PDO) for the surgical treatment of hallux valgus. Chir Organi Mov 2005;90(4):365–9.

33. Murawski DE, Beskin JL. Increased displacement maximizes the utility of the distal chevron osteotomy for hallux valgus deformity correction. Foot Ankle Int 2008;29(2):155–63.

Minimally Invasive Hallux Valgus Correction

Francesco Oliva, MD, PhD[a], Umile Giuseppe Longo, MD[b],
Nicola Maffulli, MD, MS, PhD, FRCS (Orth)[c,*]

KEYWORDS
- Minimally invasive • Hallux valgus • Percutaneous
- Bosch • Correction • Osteotomy

Many orthopedic subspecialties have embraced minimally invasive procedures. The potential advantages of minimally invasive surgery (MIS) in foot procedures mainly involve reduction in operating time and surgical trauma, the possibility of performing the procedure bilaterally, the use of distal anesthetic block, and early weight-bearing.[1] Minimum incision surgery is defined as surgery performed through the smallest incision necessary to perform the procedure properly; percutaneous surgery is defined as surgery performed within the smallest possible working incision in a closed fashion.[2] MIS, whether performed percutaneously or with minimum incision, needs dedicated instruments, and, at times, extensive use of fluoroscopy.[1] Recently, arthroscopic and endoscopic attempts to correct hallux valgus deformity have been developed.[3,4]

In 1945, Morton Polokoff performed subdermal surgery using fine instruments, such as chisels, rasps, and spears; later Leonard Britton performed percutaneous first metatarsal opening, closing, and dorsiflexion wedge osteotomies and Akin osteotomies to treat bunion deformities.[5]

MIS of the foot was first introduced in the 1970s by North American podiatrists.[6] The latest percutaneous surgical procedures are modifications of the Lamprecht-Kramer-Bosch technique described in 1982,[7–9] originally based on a Hohmann-type metatarsal subcapital linear osteotomy.[10] Isham[11] in 1991 described a minimal invasive distal metatarsal osteotomy procedure without any implants. In a recent French study, patients undergoing minimally invasive procedures for hallux valgus showed a significantly shorter hospital stay and sick leave.[12]

Percutaneous and minimum incision techniques seem to be indicated in high-risk patients who have ulceration or recurrent ulceration as a means of performing limb preservation/salvage without extensive soft tissue and osseous trauma.[13–16]

The most common complication following minimally invasive foot procedures is recurrence of the deformity, a consequence of incorrect selection of the procedure, incorrect surgical technique, and underestimated healing time of the osteotomy.[12,17,18] Scientific reports on MIS for hallux valgus correction have recently originated more from European[17,19,20] than from North American orthopedic foot surgeons.[18]

INDICATIONS

We use a minimally invasive procedure to correct a reducible hallux valgus when the hallux valgus angle (HVA) is up to 40° and the intermetatarsal angle (IMA) is up to 20°. The operation can be performed independently of congruence of the metatarsophalangeal joint, in patients who have marked increase of the distal metatarsal articular angle, and also in patients who have mild degenerative arthritis of the first metatarsophalangeal joint.

[a] Department of Orthopaedic and Trauma Surgery, University of Rome "Tor Vergata", 1, 00155 Rome, Italy
[b] Department of Orthopaedic and Trauma Surgery, University Campus Biomedico of Rome, Via Alvaro del Portillo 200, 00128 Rome, Italy
[c] Centre for Sports and Exercise Medicine, Barts and The London School of Medicine and Dentistry, Queen Mary University of London, Mile End Hospital, 275 Bancroft Road, E1 4DG London, UK
* Corresponding author.
E-mail address: n.maffulli@qmul.ac.uk (N. Maffulli).

Orthop Clin N Am 40 (2009) 525–530
doi:10.1016/j.ocl.2009.06.005
0030-5898/09/$ – see front matter © 2009 Elsevier Inc. All rights reserved.

orthopedic.theclinics.com

Contraindications include severe deformity with the intermetatarsal angle greater than 20°, severe degenerative disease or stiffness of the metatarsophalangeal joint, and severe instability of the metatarsocruciform or metatarsophalangeal joint.[20]

Magnan and colleagues suggest as indication for the percutaneous surgical correction a painful primary mild to moderate hallux valgus deformity with a first intermetatarsal angle of 10° to 20° and a hallux valgus angle of less than 40°, juvenile hallux valgus deformity with an increased distal metatarsal articular angle, and isolated hallux valgus interphalangeus deformity. These authors suggest not using this technique in patients who have a hallux rigidus and in patients in whom a previous Keller procedure has failed.[21,22] Giannini and colleagues[23,24] proposed MIS to correct mild to moderate reducible deformity when the HVA is up to 40° and the IMA is up to 20°.

SURGICAL TECHNIQUE

We originally used general anesthesia, but lately, in patients who have isolated hallux valgus deformity, we perform the procedure under local anesthesia by direct infiltration and digital nerve block. With the patient supine, the foot is prepared in the standard fashion and exsanguinated. A calf tourniquet is used. Soft tissue release is not needed, given the large lateral shift of the metatarsal head achievable. If stiffness of the metatarsophalangeal joint is present, manual stretching of the adductor hallucis is performed, forcing the hallux into a varus position before the skin incision. A 1.5- to 2-cm medial incision is made just proximal to the bunion. The incision is deepened through the skin and subcutaneous tissue, and the medial aspect of the first metatarsal is exposed. The soft tissues are retracted dorsally and plantarly. A 2-mm Kirschner wire is inserted (Fig. 1), using a drill passing through the incision into the soft tissue adjacent to the distal end of the first metatarsal and the hallux in a proximal-to-distal direction parallel to the longitudinal axis of the hallux. The Kirschner wire exits just medial to the tip of the hallux close to the nail, and is retracted up to the proximal end. An osteotomy is performed using a standard pneumatic saw with a 9.5 × 25 × 0.4-mm blade (Hall Surgical Linvatec Corporation, Largo, Florida) (Fig. 2). Using different inclinations of the bone cut and different displacements of the head (lateral, dorsal, plantar, medial tilt, or rotation), it is possible to correct each component of the deformity.

With a small osteotome, we mobilize the head of the first metatarsal. We obtain the correction by translating the metatarsal head laterally (Fig. 3).

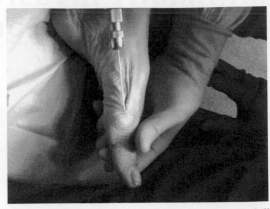

Fig. 1. A 2-mm Kirschner wire is inserted using a drill passing through the incision into the soft tissue adjacent to the distal end of the first metatarsal and the hallux in a proximal-to-distal direction parallel to the longitudinal axis of the hallux.

The osteotomy is stabilized by inserting a Kirschner wire into the medullary canal of the first metatarsal in a distal-to-proximal direction to the base of the first metatarsal (Fig. 4). After ensuring that no dorsal migration of the head of the first metatarsal had occurred, another 2-mm Kirschner wire is inserted in a proximal-to-distal and medial-to-lateral direction (Figs. 5 and 6), from the medial and dorsal aspect of the metatarsal shaft, 12 mm proximal to the subcapital osteotomy, directing it toward the head of the first metatarsal to further stabilize the osteotomy. The skin is sutured, and the protruding Kirschner wires are curved and cut. Lateral release with dissection of the lateral soft tissues is not usually performed. Recently we have slightly modified this technique, adding a second Kirschner wire, which we insert in a proximal-to-distal and medial-to-lateral direction from the shaft of the first metatarsal toward the head

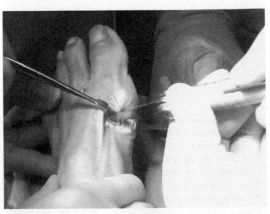

Fig. 2. An osteotomy is performed using a standard pneumatic saw.

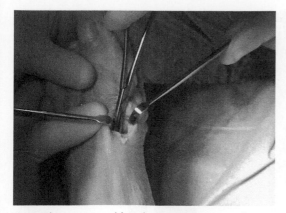

Fig. 3. The metatarsal head is translated laterally.

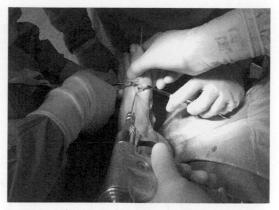

Fig. 5. Another 2-mm Kirschner wire is inserted in a proximal-to-distal and medial-to-lateral direction.

of the first metatarsal. This second Kirschner wire stabilizes the osteotomy avoiding accidental dorsal translation of the osteotomy in the early postoperative stage. We usually remove this second Kirschner wire after 2 weeks postoperatively (Fig. 7A–D).

POSTOPERATIVE MANAGEMENT

A compressive bandage is applied, and control radiographs (anteroposterior and oblique views) are obtained. Walking is allowed immediately, and the patient is advised to walk on his or her heel. We also prescribe a postoperative shoe with a flat rigid sole. Foot elevation is advised when at rest. The Kirschner wire fixation described produces elastic stabilization, favoring early healing of the osteotomy combined with early weight-bearing. We remove the remaining Kirschner wire 6 weeks after the operation in the clinic, taking plain radiographs at that stage.[20]

Cycling and swimming are encouraged. Patients are told to wear comfortable normal shoes for 3 to 6 months, gradually returning to normal footwear. Patients are reviewed 3 months after the procedure for further radiographic and clinical checks. The frequency of further follow-up appointments is variable, generally taking place at yearly intervals. Other authors remove the Kirschner wire 4 weeks after the operation and tape the hallux for 6 weeks, changing the dressing weekly. The taping should maintain the hallux in slight hypercorrection.[21]

DISCUSSION

The most common complication following foot MIS is recurrence of the deformity, attributable to an incorrect procedure selection. In the literature, mainly case series are reported, and with a marked lack of adequately planned and executed randomized studies comparing traditional open and mini-invasive surgical techniques for the correction of hallux valgus.[18] Weil[25] described complications

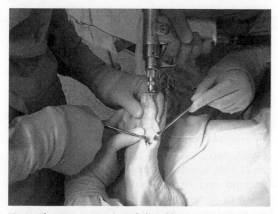

Fig. 4. The osteotomy is stabilized by inserting a Kirschner wire into the medullary canal of the first metatarsal in a distal-to-proximal direction to the base of the first metatarsal.

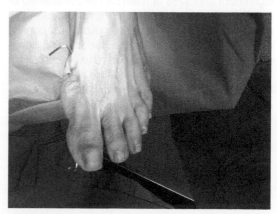

Fig. 6. The final results.

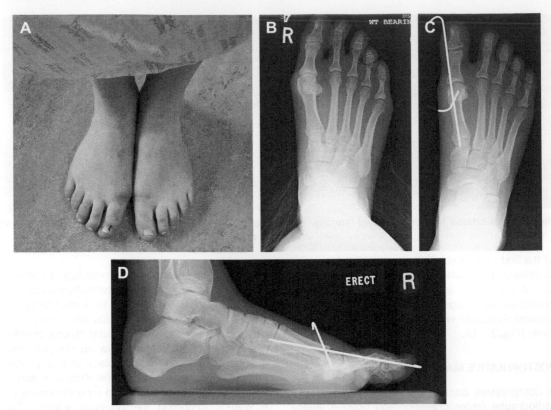

Fig. 7. A patient undergoing the double Kirschner wire technique. (*A*) Clinical picture. (*B*) Plain radiographs showing an anteroposterior view of the right foot. (*C*) Postoperative anteroposterior view. The second Kirschner wire is inserted from proximal to the osteotomy. (*D*) Postoperative lateral view showing that the main Kirschner wire is placed dorsally to the head of the metatarsal.

of minimal incision surgery, including tendon, vascular, and nerve injuries.

De Prado and colleagues[17] describes among general complications infections in 0.2% and phlebitis in 1% of patients. The same author describes shortening of the first metatarsal (100%), displacement of the osteotomy (3%), and delayed union (8%). Only 3% of osteotomy displacements are significant and 37% of them can be considered of no clinical relevance. Delayed union occurred in 8% of cases. Soft tissue complications consist mainly of skin complications related to portal placement, nerve complications, and vascular complications. Portal and skin complications are burns (3%). Complications related to nerves can be classified as transient (12%) and permanent (0.5%). Vascular complications are bleeding and hematomas, but no ischemic complications were recorded; restriction of mobility (4%) and persistent pain (3%) can be a problem for some patients.[11]

Magnan and coworkers[21] note plantar displacement or angulation occurred in 49% of their case series with dorsiflexion occurring in 12%, with a recurrence rate of 2.5% (3 of 118 feet) recorded.

Weinberger and colleagues[26] performed a retrospective review of 301 percutaneous, unfixated first metatarsal osteotomies for treating hallux valgus that revealed a mean first metatarsal shortening of 5.8 mm ± 2.6 mm, 47 dorsal malunions (15.6%), 11 infections (3.7%), 7 second metatarsal stress fractures (2.3%), 4 delayed unions (1.2%), and 1 hallux varus (0.3%).

Giannini and colleagues[23] reported only nine poor results after 4 years of follow up on 190 patients treated with MIS with an American Orthopaedic Foot and Ankle Society (AOFAS) score less than 60. Portaluri[24] performed a retrospective clinical and radiographic evaluation of 182 Bosch procedures with a mean follow-up of 16.4 ± 2.4 months. He reported eight superficial infections (4.4%), two ulcerations around the Kirschner pin site (1.1%), and two dorsal malunions (1.1%).

Sanna and Ruiu[27] performed a retrospective review of 52 feet treated with percutaneous distal first metatarsal osteotomies. Over a mean follow-up period of 31.5 months, the authors reported four (7.4%) superficial infections and three (5.8%) ulcerations around the Kirschner pin site, one

(2%) recurrent deformity, one (2%) incidence of permanent anesthesia about the hallux, and one (2%) over-lengthening of the first metatarsal.

Piqué-Vidal[28] reviewed prospectively 94 percutaneous, unfixated first metatarsal and Akin osteotomies similar to the Bosch procedure and reported four delayed unions (4.3%) and no incidences of infection, nonunion, or avascular necrosis.

De Giorgi and colleagues[29] studied 27 consecutive feet operated using Bosch technique at an average follow-up of 19 months (6 months to 5 years). They observed good results in the immediate postoperative time but all patients had worse radiographic measurements at follow-up. Nevertheless, they were clinically satisfied, and only one nonunion was recorded.

After 98 percutaneous distal osteotomies of the first metatarsal with a mean follow-up of 76.2 months, Baietta and colleagues[30] reported a mean score AOFAS of 89.9, with 96% of the patients satisfied. They recorded only four superficial infections around the Kirschner wire, two recurrences of hallux valgus, one hallux rigidus, and five cases of metatarsalgia.

Recently, an arthroscopy-assisted hallux valgus deformity correction with percutaneous screw fixation has been reported. Of 94 feet treated with this technique just 2 experienced symptomatic recurrence and were submitted to a revision operation.[4]

The only randomized trial planned to recruit 20 patients in each arm of the study.[18] The authors experienced so many problems with the minimally invasive procedure that they had to stop the trial and abandon the minimally invasive technique. Examining that report, it is evident that although the authors were extremely experienced with the traditional technique, they included in their study all the patients in whom MIS had been planned. Their results could therefore be biased because they had not come out of the learning curve yet. In addition, they did not follow the original description of the MIS technique, and they completed the osteotomy by blunt instruments. Finally, they used 1.6-mm instead of 2-mm Kirschner wires for fixation, thus markedly decreasing the stiffness of the stabilization, making the distal capital fragment more prone to fixation. Also, by imparting less stiffness to the osteotomy, they may have inadvertently increased time to healing, making it more likely for recurrence of the deformity to occur after removal of the Kirschner wire.

In our case series of 15 consecutive female patients, we reported no major complications and no recurrence after 2 years of follow-up.[20] González and colleagues[31] hypothesized that the healing

time of the osteotomy can be shorter than with traditional techniques for two basic reasons: (1) the minimal injury to vessels and surrounding soft tissues caused by the minimally invasive technique, and (2) the bone detritus ("bone mush") at the osteotomy site from the use of cutting burs and reaming the bunion may behave as an autologous bone graft to stimulate healing of the osteotomy.

We usually remove the proximal Kirschner wire after 2 weeks and the main Kirschner wire after 6 weeks. We acknowledge that this may expose the patients to superficial infections, but the transverse osteotomy will likely require this time to heal.

In conclusion, if the indications are adequate, and provided that dedicated instruments, sufficient technical capability, and enough care are used during the learning curve, MIS is a suitable surgical choice for correction of uncomplicated hallux valgus deformity.[6] Adequately powered and accurately performed randomized prospective clinical trials are needed in this field.

REFERENCES

1. David C, Sammarco G, James G. Minimum incision surgery. Foot Ankle Int 1992;13(3):157–60.
2. Van Enoo RE, Cane EM. Minimal incision surgery: a plastic technique or a cover-up? Clin Podiatr Med Surg 1986;3(2):321–35.
3. Lui TH, Ng S, Chan KB. Endoscopic distal soft tissue procedure in hallux valgus surgery. Arthroscopy 2005;21:1403 e1–7.
4. Lui TH, Chan KB, Chow HT, et al. Arthroscopy-assisted correction of hallux valgus deformity. Arthroscopy 2008;24(8):875–80.
5. Hymes L. Introduction: brief history of the use of minimum incision surgery (MIS). In: Fielding MD, editor. Forefoot minimum incision in podiatric medicine: a handbook on primary corrective procedures on the human foot using minimum incisions with minimum trauma. New York: Futura Pub Co; 1977. p. 1–2.
6. De Lavigne C, Guillo S, Laffenêtre O, et al. The treatment of hallux valgus with the mini-invasive technique. Interact Surg 2007;2:31–7.
7. Bösch P, Markowski H, Rannicher V. Technik und erste Ergebnisse der subkutanen distalen Metatarsale-I-Osteotomie. Orthop Praxis 1990;26:51–6 [in German].
8. Hohmann G. Symptomatische oder physiologische Behandlung des Hallux valgus. Münch Med Wochenschr 1921;68:1042–5 [in German].
9. Lamprecht E, Kramer J. Die Metatarsale-I-Osteotomie nach Kramer zur Behandlung des Hallux valgus. Orthop Prax 1982;28:635–45 [in German].
10. Bösch P, Wanke S, Legenstein R. Hallux valgus correction by the method of Bösch: a new technique

with a seven-to-ten year follow-up. Foot Ankle Clin 2000;5:485–98.

11. Isham SA. The Reverdin-Isham procedure for the correction of hallux abducto valgus. A distal metatarsal osteotomy procedure. Clin Podiatr Med Surg 1991;8:81–94.

12. Leemrijse T, Valtin B, Besse JL. [Hallux valgus surgery in 2005. Conventional, mini-invasive or percutaneous surgery? Uni- or bilateral? Hospitalisation or one-day surgery?]. Rev Chir Orthop Reparatrice Appar Mot 2008;94:111–27 [in French].

13. Roukis TS. Central metatarsal head–neck osteotomies: indications and operative techniques. Clin Podiatr Med Surg 2005;22(2):197–222.

14. Roukis TS. The tailor's bunionette deformity: a field guide to surgical correction. Clin Podiatr Med Surg 2005;22(2):223–45.

15. Weitzel S, Trnka HJ, Petroutsas J. Transverse medial slide osteotomy for bunionette deformity: long-term results. Foot Ankle Int 2007;28(7):794–8.

16. Roukis TS, Schade VL. Minimum-incision metatarsal osteotomies. Clin Podiatr Med Surg 2008;25:587–607.

17. De Prado M, Ripoll PL, Vaquero J, et al. Tratamiento quirurgico per cutaneo del hallux mediante osteotomias multiples. Rev Orthop Traumatol 2003;47:406–16 [in Spanish].

18. Kadakia AR, Smerek JP, Myerson MS. Radiographic results after percutaneous distal metatarsal osteotomy for correction of hallux valgus deformity. Foot Ankle Int 2007;28:355–60.

19. De Prado M, Ripoll PL, Golano P. Cirurgia percutanea del pie. Barcelona: Ed. Masson; 2003. [in Spanish].

20. Maffulli N, Oliva F, Coppola C, et al. Minimally invasive hallux valgus correction: a technical note and a feasibility study. J Surg Orthop Adv 2005;14:193–8.

21. Magnan B, Bortolazzi R, Samaila E, et al. Percutaneous distal metatarsal osteotomy for correction of hallux valgus. Surgical technique. J Bone Joint Surg Am 2006;88:135–48.

22. Magnan B, Samaila E, Viola G, et al. Minimally invasive retrocapital osteotomy of the first metatarsal in hallux valgus deformity. Oper Orthop Traumatol 2008;20:89–96.

23. Giannini S, Vannini F, Faldini C, et al. The minimally invasive hallux valgus correction (S.E.R.I.). Interact Surg 2007;2:17–23.

24. Portaluri M. Hallux valgus correction by the method of Bosch: a clinical evaluation. Foot Ankle Clin 2000;5(3):499–511.

25. Weil LS. Minimal invasive surgery of the foot and ankle. J Foot Ankle Surg 2001;40:61.

26. Weinberger BH, Fulp JM, Falstrom P, et al. Retrospective evaluation of percutaneous bunionectomies and distal osteotomies without internal fixation. Clin Podiatr Med Surg 1991;8(1):111–36.

27. Sanna P, Ruiu GA. Percutaneous distal osteotomy of the first metatarsal (PDO) for the surgical treatment of hallux valgus. Chir Organi Mov 2005;90(4):365–9.

28. Piqué-Vidal C. The effect of temperature elevation during discontinuous use of rotator burrs in the correction of hallux valgus. J Foot Ankle Surg 2005;44(5):336–44.

29. De Giorgi S, Mascolo V, Losito A. The correction of hallux valgus by Bösch tecnique (PDO - Percutaneus Distal Osteotomy). GIOT 2003;29:161–4.

30. Baietta D, Perusi M, Cassini M. [Hallux valgus surgical treatment with Bosch technique: clinical evaluation and surgical consideration after 5 years]. GIOT 2007;33:107–13.

31. González-Lahoz J, Rodríguez RS, Cadena ML. Functional, esthetic and radiographic results of treatment of hallux valgus with minimally invasive surgery. Acta Ortop Mex 2005;19:42–6.

From Mini-Invasive to Non-Invasive Treatment Using Monopolar Radiofrequency: The Next Orthopaedic Frontier

Terry L. Whipple, MD

KEYWORDS
- Radiofrequency • Tendinopathy • Sprains
- Non-invasive • Inflammation • Anti-nociceptive

RADIOFREQUENCY

Radiofrequency (RF) was first introduced to the field of neurology in the nineteenth century.[1] RF energy is currently the most commonly used energy source to generate therapeutic levels of heat. Supraphysiologic temperature has been used medically to produce structural and biologic responses in tissue. In orthopaedics, the main target of supraphysiologic temperatures is collagen-based connective tissue. Although most commonly used as an ablative fine focus (electrocautery) tool, it is possible to use radiofrequency in a nonablative form for controlled heating of target tissues for structural and biologic therapeutic effects.

STRUCTURAL EFFECTS
Collagen Connective Tissue

Heating collagen with RF energy is time-dependent. At temperatures of $60°C$, the long sequences of the hydrogen bonds that stabilize the triple helix of collagen molecules[2] break, which collapses the molecule and causes soft connective tissue to shrink. The linear collagen fibers of the tissue are coagulated, as appreciated on light microscopy and with polarized light. The process has been used to shrink and tighten joint capsule tissue and ligaments in a predictable fashion (**Fig. 1**).

Nociceptors

The actual symptoms of tendinopathy may arise from biochemical agents that irritate nociceptors.[3] Takahashi and colleagues[4] studied the antinociceptive effects of RF: bipolar RF induced acute degeneration and ablation of sensory nerve fibers. There is also a delayed regrowth of nociceptive afferent fibers into irradiated tissues. This afferent denervation produces an antinociceptive effect in treated tissues and forms the basis for the clinical use of RF in pain management.

BIOLOGIC EFFECTS OF RADIOFREQUENCY

At temperatures above $60°C$, there is a predictable influx of macrophages and other inflammatory cells. These cells produce heat shock proteins. Supraphysiologic temperatures induce an overexpression of heat shock proteins.[5] These proteins protect cells in vivo and in vitro against a variety of insults.[6–9] Wound healing responses (WHRs) of surgical and thermal injuries follow a predictable cascade of inflammatory events. Using RF to irradiate tissues to heat them to supraphysiologic temperatures induces a predictable inflammatory response similar in time and nature to the WHR.

EFFECT ON TENDONS AND LIGAMENTS

The histopathologic lesion of tendinopathy is a failed WHR. In 1979, Nirschl described the

American Self Orthopaedics, Orthopaedic Research of Virginia, Richmond, VA 23233, USA
E-mail address: whipple@americanself.com

Orthop Clin N Am 40 (2009) 531–535
doi:10.1016/j.ocl.2009.06.006

ATFL Treated
Left H&E Stain--Right same under polarized light

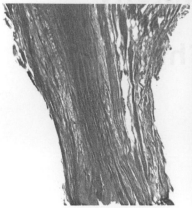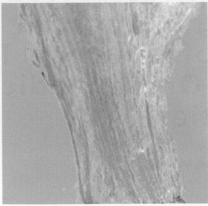

Fig. 1. Section of mcRF treated human ATFL.

histopathologic findings of 88 elbows treated operatively for tennis elbow and reported immature fibroblastic and vascular infiltration[10] known as myxoid degeneration, "the result of failed tendon healing."[11] Cellular hallmarks of inflammation were notably absent. Common problems of tendons and ligaments (eg, tennis elbow, golfer's elbow, and patellar and Achilles tendinopathy) are noninflammatory conditions. Given the lack of inflammation, anti-inflammatory therapeutic options, including nonsteroidal anti-inflammatory drugs and corticosteroids, are contraindicated.[12] Preclinical and clinical studies have demonstrated the benefit of inducing an appropriate WHR for the management of tendinopathy.[13–18]

Ligament injuries are common and debilitating musculoskeletal injuries. Conservative management protocols have remained essentially unchanged for decades. Despite ice, compression, elevation, and splinting of acute ligament injuries, still some 40% of acute ankle sprains, for example, remain functionally unstable and susceptible to reinjury. Treatment of injured

ligaments with radiofrequency physically shortens the elongated structural fibers, which improves stability of the joints they span.

EFFECT ON MUSCLE

The effect of RF on muscle is mediated by the impact on myogenic precursor cells and is emerging as an effective treatment for some blunt trauma muscle injuries.[19] RF stimulates the production of myogenic precursor cells for muscle tissue repair and replacement, simultaneously inducing the inflammatory cascade necessary to remove hemorrhage remnants and produce an antinociceptive response.

Noninvasive Monopolar Capacitive-coupled Radiofrequency

Noninvasive monopolar capacitive-coupled RF (mcRF) is made possible by the production of a reverse thermal gradient and capacitive coupling the energy into a volume of tissue (**Fig. 2**).

Reverse Thermal Gradient

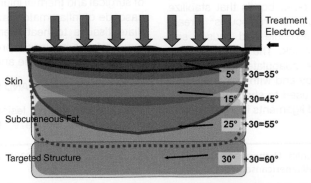

Fig. 2. Conceptual illustration of Reverse Thermal Gradient protecting superficial structures from mcRF heat.

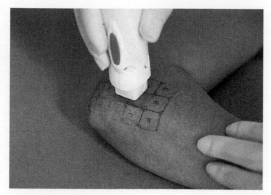

Fig. 3. Sequencing grid for treatment field for lateral epicondylitis.

Monopolar Capacitive-coupled Radiofrequency in Orthopaedics

When used in orthopaedics, noninvasive mcRF cools down a volume of tissue while producing an energy field with a greater depth of penetration only possible via a capacitive coupled electrode. Noninvasive mcRF for the treatment of conditions of ligaments and tendons benefits from the three main mechanisms of action of RF: the ability of the collagen to reach a contracted phase, the antinociceptive effect, and the ability to stimulate the WHR.

PRECLINICAL AND CLINICAL BACKGROUND

Studies were performed using cadaveric elbow and ankle specimens.[20] Pretreatment dissections isolated specific target structures (the tendon of extensor carpi radialis brevis in the elbow, and the anterior talofibular ligament in the ankle) and fiber thermal sensors were implanted. The target tissues were treated with mcRF (Alpha Orthopaedics, Hayward, CA) while recording the thermal effect in the target tissues to ensure they reached and maintained the critical 60°C threshold level. The extensor carpi radialis brevis and anterior talofibular ligament were then harvested and examined under light, polarized light, and electron microscopy. mcRF delivered percutaneously is capable of denaturing the collagen molecules within superficial ligaments and tendons without damaging the overlying skin or subcutaneous layers (**Fig. 3**).[20] In vivo, the resulting WHRs from a thermal injury from noninvasive mcRF are similar in nature and timing to those of incisional or burn wounds.[21]

THE SYSTEM

The Alpha Orthopaedics' AT2 System is a noninvasive mcRF device. The generator supplies RF power while continuously monitoring and displaying output current, output energy, treatment duration, and measured impedance (**Fig. 4**). The handpiece assembly is fitted with a monopolar RF electrode, which is equipped with four thermistors to cool the skin and subcutaneous tissue during treatment and a memory chip to record skin temperature and prevent thermal injury.

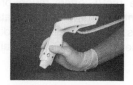

Electrode & Handpiece

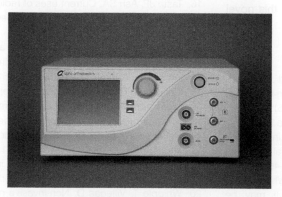

Radiofrequency Generator

Fig. 4. Alpha AT2 mcRF system. (*Courtesy of* Alpha Orthopaedics, Hayward, CA; with permission.)

DISCUSSION

Sprains, strains, and tendinopathies are common musculoskeletal injuries. The economic burden on the workplace from incapacitation and absenteeism because of these injuries is immense. Traditional conservative treatment has changed little in the past several decades. Anti-inflammatory medications are counterproductive and, in fact, actually delay the natural healing response. Nonsteroidal anti-inflammatory drugs have potentially negative effects during the proliferative phase of healing because they are associated with decreased DNA synthesis.[22] Clinical outcomes after corticosteroid injections for tendinopathies are worse than placebo at 26 and 52 weeks.[23,24] In most instances, a controlled inflammatory response after ligament and tendon injuries is desirable.

RF surgical treatment of recalcitrant tennis elbow lesions provided earlier pain relief and better grip strength in a randomized trial compared with extensor carpi radialis brevis tendon release or repair.[14] Recently, a noninvasive mcRF technology that is capable of delivering high levels of RF energy in a noninvasive fashion was introduced. The bases of the clinical application of the technology are its ability to raise the temperatures of tendons and ligaments to a point at which collagen structures denature[20] and its ability to trigger an effective WHR.[25] Other RF generators used for this purpose, most of which are bipolar electrodes, require an open or otherwise invasive surgical procedure to access the injured structures. Noninvasive mcRF offers a therapeutic alternative to the noninvasive standard of care.

SUMMARY

Noninvasive mcRF offers much promise in the management of common tendinopathies and ligament injuries. Additional clinical studies are necessary to understand the full potential of this novel technology.

REFERENCES

1. Cosman ER, Nashold BS, Ovelman-Levitt J. Theoretical aspects of radiofrequency lesions in the dorsal root entry zone. Neurosurgery 1984;15(6):945–50.
2. Miles CA, Burjanadze TV, Bailey AJ. The kinetics of the thermal denaturation of collagen in unrestrained rat tail tendon determined by differential scanning calorimetry. J Mol Biol 1995;245(4):437–46.
3. Khan KM, Cook JL, Maffulli N, et al. Where is the pain coming from in tendinopathy? It may be biochemical, not only structural, in origin. Br J Sports Med 2000;34(2):81–3.
4. Takahashi N, Tasto JP, Ritter M, et al. Pain relief through an antinociceptive effect after radiofrequency application. Am J Sports Med 2007;35(5):805–10.
5. Yang S. Le traitement de choc thermique augmente la survie des myoblastes porcins après transplantation autologue dans le muscle squelettique. Geneve: Faculté de Médecine; Section de Médecine Clinique; Département de chirurgie; Service de chirurgie orthopédique et de traumatologie de l'appareil moteur, Université de Génève; 2005 [in French].
6. Fink AL. Chaperone-mediated protein folding. Physiol Rev 1999;79(2):425–49.
7. Jaattela M. Heat shock proteins as cellular lifeguards. Ann Med 1999;31(4):261–71.
8. Sharp FR, Massa SM, Swanson RA. Heat-shock protein protection. Trends Neurosci 1999;22(3):97–9.
9. Williams RS, Thomas JA, Fina M, et al. Human heat shock protein 70 (hsp70) protects murine cells from injury during metabolic stress. J Clin Invest 1993;92(1):503–8.
10. Nirschl RP, Pettrone FA. Tennis elbow: the surgical treatment of lateral epicondylitis. J Bone Joint Surg Am 1979;61(6A):832–9.
11. Kraushaar BS, Nirschl RP. Tendinosis of the elbow (tennis elbow): clinical features and findings of histological, immunohistochemical, and electron microscopy studies. J Bone Joint Surg Am 1999;81(2):259–78.
12. Magra M, Maffulli N. Nonsteroidal antiiflammatory drugs in tendinopathy: friend or foe. Clin J Sport Med 2006;16(1):1–3.
13. Amiel D, Ball ST, Tasto JP. Chondrocyte viability and metabolic activity after treatment of bovine articular cartilage with bipolar radiofrequency: an in vitro study. Arthroscopy 2004;20(5):503–10.
14. Meknas K, Odden-Miland A, Mercer JB, et al. Radiofrequency microtenotomy: a promising method for treatment of recalcitrant lateral epicondylitis. Am J Sports Med 2008;36(10):1960–5.
15. Tasto JP. The role of radiofrequency-based devices in shaping the future of orthopedic surgery. Orthopedics 2006;29(10):874–5.
16. Tasto JP, Ash SA. Current uses of radiofrequency in arthroscopic knee surgery. Am J Knee Surg 1999; 12(3):186–91.
17. Tasto JP, Cummings J, Medlock V, et al. Microtenotomy using a radiofrequency probe to treat lateral epicondylitis. Arthroscopy 2005;21(7):851–60.
18. Taverna E, Battistella F, Sansone V, et al. Radiofrequency-based plasma microtenotomy compared with arthroscopic subacromial decompression yields equivalent outcomes for rotator cuff tendinosis. Arthroscopy 2007;23(10):1042–51.
19. Hayashi A. Getting athletes back in the game: a global view. AAOS Now 2008;2(10):1–6.
20. Whipple T, Villegas D. Non-invasive monopolar radiofrequency energy for the treatment of tendons and ligaments: Temperatures achieved and

histological outcomes. Richmond (VA): Orthopaedic Research of Virginia; 2009.

21. Bernstein L. Tendinosis of the shoulder. Miss Valley Med J 1951;73(6):155–7.

22. Almekinders LC, Banes AJ, Bracey LW. An in vitro investigation into the effects of repetitive motion and nonsteroidal anti-inflammatory medication on human tendon fibroblasts. Am J Sports Med 1995; 23(1):119–23.

23. Bisset L, Smidt N, Van der Windt DA, et al. Conservative treatments for tennis elbow: do subgroups of patients respond differently? Rheumatology 2007; 46(10):1601–5.

24. Bjordal JM, Lopes-Martins R, Joensen J, et al. A systematic review with procedural assessments and metaanalysis of low level laser therapy in lateral elbow tendinopathy (tennis elbow). BMC Musculoskelet Disord 2008;9:75 (10):1186/1471-2474-1189-1175.

25. England LJ, Egbert BM, Pope K. Dermal wound healing in an animal model following monopolar radiofrequency treatment. Presented at the Wound Healing Society Meeting. Chicago (IL), May 18–21, 2005.

Minimally Invasive Computer-Navigated Total Knee Arthroplasty

Nicola Biasca, MD[a],*, Thomas-Oliver Schneider, MD[b], Matthias Bungartz, MD[a]

KEYWORDS

- Computer-assisted navigated surgery
- Total knee arthroplasty • Malalignment • Malrotation
- Minimally invasive surgery

Total knee arthroplasty (TKA) is a highly successful procedure, with long-term follow-up studies reporting clinical success rates of 72% to 100%, as evaluated by pain reduction, functional improvement, and overall patient satisfaction at 10 to 20 years' follow-up.[1–5] Although TKA is generally successful, and despite the advances in the surgical techniques, instrumentation, and implant designs, between 5% and 8% of all patients develop complications such as anterior knee pain, loosening, instability, malpositioning, infection, or fractures.[6–8] The success of TKA depends on several factors, including patient selection, pre-operative deformity, appropriate implant design, correct surgical technique, soft tissue balancing, and alignment of the limb. Correct alignment of implanted components is considered one important factor that is under the surgeon's control at surgery. There is a definite relationship between the accuracy of implant positioning and longevity.[9–22] The most common cause of revision TKA is error in surgical technique: small changes in component positioning can lead to significant changes in post-operative performance.[23] Imperfections in the axial alignment of the femoral and tibial components, imperfect rotational alignment, improper ligament balancing, and incorrect joint-line restoration can lead to soft tissue imbalance and an inability to re-establish optimal kinematics and the overall

biomechanics of the joint, with persistent anterior knee pain, patellar maltracking, varus/valgus instability, or limitation of movement.[9–14,23]

To address the problem of correct alignment, various mechanical alignment guides are used to improve the precision of implant positioning, but technical errors in surgical alignment still occur. Surgical navigation systems help reduce errors in component alignment during TKA. Although knee navigation systems are not yet universally accepted, several investigators have demonstrated with conventional radiography and CT that TKA implanted using computer-assisted navigation has more accurate component alignment than TKA implanted conventionally.[9,23–30]

Patient demand, potential health care savings, and the development of new instrumentation and techniques have led to rapid advances in less invasive surgical approaches. Minimally invasive surgical (MIS) approaches have been used with success in numerous types of surgical procedures, both arthroscopic and open. The introduction of MIS approaches for TKA has been driven partially by the use of small incisions and minimal soft tissue approaches in the performance of unicompartmental knee arthroplasty.[31,32] Motivating factors for patients include a possible reduction in duration of hospitalization and costs as well as concerns about post-operative pain, prolonged and

[a] Clinics of Orthopedic Surgery, Sports Medicine and Trauma Surgery, Department of Surgery, Spital Oberengadin, CH-7503, Samedan (St. Moritz), Switzerland
[b] Department of Orthopaedics, Hirslanden Clinic Permanence, CH-3018, Bern, Switzerland
* Corresponding author.
E-mail addresses: Biasca@medicmotion.com (N. Biasca); http://www.orthopaedie-samedan.ch

Orthop Clin N Am 40 (2009) 537–563
doi:10.1016/j.ocl.2009.06.007
0030-5898/09/$ – see front matter © 2009 Elsevier Inc. All rights reserved.

arduous rehabilitation, and less-than-ideal functional outcomes associated with conventional TKA. Minimally invasive knee arthroplasty techniques (MIS TKA) also have been marketed intensively by the orthopedic implant industry. There is, however, concern about loss of accuracy in implant placement and increased complications related to skin slough and infection when a minimally invasive approach is used.[33,34]

Proponents of MIS TKA report that, compared with patients undergoing conventional TKA, patients undergoing MIS TKA experience decreased blood loss, shortened hospital stay, less need for pain-control medications, and faster recovery of knee range of motion, all without compromise of accuracy or short-term outcome.[35–37] Critics believe that the disadvantages include reduced operative visualization, a steep learning curve, an increased risk of complications, excessive skin trauma, and compromised implant fixation and alignment. Some surgeons have expressed concerns about the use of MIS TKA and the safety of operations performed "through a keyhole" and argue that at present there is no credible evidence that smaller incisions significantly benefit the patient receiving MIS TKA. Also, because of the steep learning curve, MIS TKA should not be performed unless the surgeon has a high-volume arthroplasty practice.[38,39] Although several recent studies demonstrate improved early clinical outcomes with the use of minimally invasive approaches, surgeons still are cautious about embracing MIS approaches, preferring a standard technique that provides consistently good clinical outcomes.[35,37,40–42] Furthermore, two recent studies reported that good alignment of TKA correlates with better clinical function, improved quality of life, quicker rehabilitation, and earlier hospital discharge.[43,44]

Here the author describes his technique of minimally invasive computer-navigated total knee arthroplasty (MIS CN-TKA) and his experience comparing two groups of patients treated with conventional computer-navigated total knee arthroplasty (CN-TKA) and MIS CN-TKA.

INDICATIONS AND CONTRAINDICATIONS FOR MINIMALLY INVASIVE COMPUTER-NAVIGATED TOTAL KNEE ARTHROPLASTY

Indications for MIS CN-TKA are similar to indications for conventional TKA: failure of nonoperative management of knee pain, loss of motion, and deformity and limitation of function resulting from arthritis.

The contraindications for MIS CN-TKA are not yet well defined; they may include patients who

have active infections, neurologic deficits, malignancies, a stiff or arthrodesed hip or ankle, extreme adiposity, extreme knee deformities, severe bone or soft tissue trauma, severe bone destruction after rheumatoid arthritis, severe contracture or reduced of range of motion, severe osteoporosis, risk factors for wound healing complications, and revision surgery of a previous implanted TKA.

SURGICAL APPROACHES FOR MINIMALLY INVASIVE TOTAL KNEE ARTHROPLASTY

The clinical definition and criteria for MIS have not been firmly established. Different parameters have been used to define MIS, including length of incision, location of incision, muscle-sparing approaches, reduced in-patient hospital stay, and rapid muscle recovery. The most definitive characteristics of MIS, which include reduced soft tissue trauma and improved post-operative functional recovery, often are overlooked.

MIS TKA uses skin incisions 8 to 12 cm long in the smallest and largest patients, respectively, compared with incision lengths of up to 25 cm in conventional approaches. The length of the skin incision is adjusted according to the surgeon's experience, the size of the implant needed, and the elasticity of the soft tissue. The length of the skin incision has only cosmetic implications and should not affect recovery. Insufficient tension on the skin may jeopardize wound healing and cause necrosis or lacerations. Although a small incision seems desirable to many patients, a small incision is not the reason these operations may have better outcomes. The minimization of soft tissue dissection and disruption, lack of patella eversion, and in situ bone-cutting techniques to minimize articular dislocation are clearly more important in producing improved outcomes. Therefore, the skin incision should not compromise the integrity of the wound or the ability to perform proper surgery with the computer-navigation technique.

The minimal incision technique can be viewed as part of a continuum in the transition from classic, more extensive exposures to the true quadriceps-sparing MIS TKA. The intention is to reduce surgical dissection without compromising the procedure. Although it often is suggested that one or another "minimally invasive" approach compromises the extensor mechanism, in truth, each of these approaches preserves the extensor mechanism to a greater degree than a standard approach.

Several approaches have been described for MIS TKA.[33,35,40,45–48] One minimally invasive technique, the minimally invasive medial parapatellar approach, simply shortens the standard quadriceps incision through a 10- to 14-cm skin incision along the anterior midline, extending from the superior pole of the patella to the superior aspect of the tubercle. The arthrotomy extends 2 to 4 cm into the quadriceps tendon proximal to the superior pole of the patella.[40,45] This approach generally enables lateral patellar subluxation, without eversion, and in many patients the exposure of critical landmarks is unimpeded. If necessary, the arthrotomy can be extended easily to a more traditional approach by gradually lengthening the incision into the quadriceps tendon.

Two alternative approaches are the modified minimally invasive subvastus approach introduced by Hofmann and colleagues[46] and the minimally invasive midvastus approach introduced by Engh and colleagues,[47] both of which reduce post-operative pain, preserve vascularity of the patella, improve patellar tracking, enhance return of quadriceps strength, decrease blood loss, and accelerate rehabilitation, even through a standard incision. With the minimally invasive subvastus approach, the capsular incision is performed entirely distal to the patellar attachment of the quadriceps mechanism. The extensor mechanism is visualized, and the medial capsular incision is made from the border of the middle of the patella along the medial side of the patellar tendon and distal to the tibial tubercle. The attachment of the muscle to the quadriceps tendon and the upper patellar bone is left intact. After a synovial release of the suprapatellar pouch is performed, and the vastus medialis obliquus (VMO) is released from the intramuscular septum, the patella can be everted or subluxed laterally. The concern with this approach is the possibility of injuring the descending genicular artery and its branches, the saphenous nerve, and intramuscular septal arteries as well as the femoral vessel as they pass through the adductor hiatus.[46] The minimally invasive midvastus approach, an excellent alternative, evolved as a compromise between the exposure of medial parapatellar approach and the benefits of the subvastus approach involving the extensor mechanism.[47] The minimally invasive midvastus approach is performed through a standard anterior midline skin incision from 3 cm above the patella and 3 cm distal to the joint line, and a medial subfascial flap is developed to expose the broad insertion of the vastus medialis (**Fig. 1**).

Extension of the intermuscular interval is facilitated by blunt finger dissection or controlled release by electrocautery. To allow full eversion of the patella, the capsular folds of the suprapatellar pouch must be release proximal to the patella.

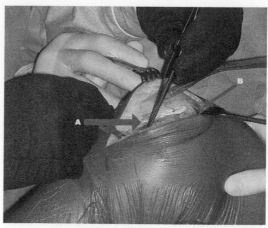

Fig. 1. The minimally invasive MIS midvastus approach. After the incision of the skin and subcutaneous tissues, the medial arthrotomy (A) is performed with an incision of the retinaculum patellae (*thick red arrow*) along the medial side of the patella to the inferior aspect of the wound. With the knee in flexion, the full thickness of the vastus medialis muscle (B) is divided in line with its muscle fibers, starting at the superomedial corner of the patella and extending proximally for about 4 to 5 cm. The amount of release is titrated later with gradual and purposeful patellar eversion and knee flexion.

The distal capsular portion of this approach involves incising the medial retinaculum and capsule along the patella and patellar tendon. This approach allows adequate exposure of the joint and improved post-operative recovery and pain relief. in an attempt to minimize soft tissue damage and preserve quadriceps muscle function, Seyler and colleagues[48] described a new approach, the minimally invasive direct lateral approach. Instruments and implants were not customized for this approach, however, and a significant rate of early complications may limit the potential of this approach until further refinements increase clinical success and make this technique suitable for general use.

Although the approaches are well recognized, these techniques often are demanding and require appropriate technical tuition even for experienced knee surgeons. The most important aspects of minimally invasive TKA are related to the soft tissues. Therefore, a cadaver course is recommended to practice the techniques of maximizing visualization using flexion, midflexion, and extension windows and of using the space produced in this fashion after each bone resection. (Further information on the author and his colleagues' cadaver course can be found at www.orthopae die-samedan.ch).

COMPUTER-ASSISTED ORTHOPEDIC SURGERY

The principle of computer-assisted orthopedic surgery is simple. A digital image serves as a map for each particular step of the procedure. This image guides the surgeon through the operation. Information from three sources can be used to establish the digital map. The first source of information is pre-operative imaging; anatomic information is collected before operation by a CT scan or MRI. The patient and the health care system are exposed to the inconvenience and cost of the CT or MRI. The second source of information is perioperative imaging, performed in the operating suite at the time of surgery. This imaging requires a specially modified fluoroscopy unit and entails the maneuvering of a relatively bulky and expensive apparatus during surgery. These two sources comprise the "image-based systems." The third information system is image free and relies on information acquired during surgery. This system allows the surgeon to quantify data, to have dynamic intraoperative feedback, and to obtain more reproducible results. A very important attribute of image-free navigation is its ability to provide instant feedback regarding in vivo kinematics of the joint. Alignment and ligament stability can be assessed with the trial components in place to ensure proper function. Furthermore, this system allows the measurement of any degree of flexion, the coronal deformity, alignment, stability, rotation, and translation. This characteristic of the navigation system provides the unique opportunity to assess in vivo kinematics of the knee during surgery and to implement beneficial changes such as refinements in soft tissue tensioning, rotational adjustment of the components, or changes in components selection.

The Stryker Leibinger Knee Navigation System (software version 3.0, Stryker-Leibinger GmbH & Co. KG, Freiburg, Germany) is an image-free navigation system that has been modified progressively since 1999 to translate the generated data more clearly for the surgeon. This system now is available in an active wireless personal computer–based guidance system, which is based on an imageless navigation method and thus does not require pre-operative CT or intraoperative fluoroscopy. It comprises a module for analyzing the alignment of the leg, the alignment of the resection planes, and thus the alignment of the prosthetic components. The system also quantifies the kinematics of the knee. Two hardware platforms are available: a laptop and a workstation version. Both are portable units consisting of a personal computer, an infrared camera system, a flat-screen monitor, and menu prompts.

The operational aspect of the system occupies a spherical area with a radius of about 50 cm. The system is most accurate when located 1.5 m from the operating field. The working space of the system is a sphere 1.0 m in diameter, so the maximum working distance is 2.0 m. The system's software runs on a standard laptop (Dell Latitude, Dell Computer Corporation, Round Rock, Texas) using Microsoft Windows 2000 (Microsoft Corporation, Redmond, Washington). The wireless navigation instruments and the camera communicate via active battery-powered light-emitting diodes. The surgeon navigates the procedure via a menu on a flat screen using a specially developed pointer. The pointer allows the surgeon to maintain control of all software functions during the procedure and to access to various submenus without using foot pedals or touching the screen. The technology does not need a computer specialist at hand. The active wireless localizers, the trackers, are fixed on special pins, which are placed at two locations bi-cortically on the distal femur and proximal tibia. The tracker's "quick connect and release" design allows simple removal of the device while maintaining precise positioning. All trackers are placed in the usual surgical field. The infrared camera registers the absolute motion in the coordinate system, and the software calculates the relative motion of two adjacent trackers. (Further details about the Stryker Knee Navigation System are available at http://www.europe.stryker.com/.)

COMPUTER-ASSISTED TOTAL KNEE ARTHROPLASTY

After standard preparation and draping, the leg is exsanguinated in a routine fashion, and the tourniquet is inflated. The procedure is initiated by positioning two femoral pins through stab wounds along the iliotibial tract and a single tibial pin distal to the tibial tuberosity. Special antirotational fixation pins have been developed specifically for this purpose that are suitable for bi-cortical anchorage and for quick connection to the trackers. The joint kinematics can be monitored whether the joint capsule is open or not. To set up the Navigation Software Setup System, the patient's data are entered, and the pointer and trackers are initialized. The anatomic landmarks then are defined with the anatomic mapping following the information from the screen. The on-screen instructions guide the surgeon. The exact center of the femoral head is pinpointed by rotational calculation with a special algorithm of the customized software. Calibration involves moving the leg to obtain various hip positions. Then single-point digitalization with the pointer is used to mark the surgical epicondylar axis, the Whiteside line, the femoral and tibial centers, and the malleoli. An algorithm of the Stryker system calculates the center of the ankle by digitalizing the malleoli. The actual pathologic deformity is calculated from the data, and the pre-operative deformities present are shown. The mechanical axis of the limb and the transepicondylar axis of the femur, the morphology of the femoral condyles, the morphology of the tibial plateau, and the long axis of the tibia are all identified, and the image data are stored. The specific anatomic landmarks and vectors recorded on the femur are the surgical medial and lateral epicondyles, the center of the distal femoral condyles, and the trochlear groove (eg, the Whiteside line). The algorithms provided by the system to determine the axial rotation of the femur average the readings of the transepicondylar axis and the Whiteside line. Surface digitalization identifies the femoral condyles and tibial plateau to determine the exact level of resection and to prevent alteration of the joint line. The data collected are used to calculate the current clinical status by mathematical algorithms, and the deformities detected pre-operatively are imaged. Kinematic curves are generated based on the distance between the landmarks during maneuvers such as varus/valgus, rotational stress, or anteroposterior movement. After the multiple landmarks have been digitalized and after the initial kinematics curves and axis have been analyzed by moving the limb from maximal extension to maximal flexion, bone cuts are performed based on the information obtained from the navigation system.

SURGICAL TECHNIQUES
Operating Theater

No specific modifications to the operative setting are needed for the procedure. A standard operating-room table with two distal foot supports allows the knee to be flexed to 45° or 90°, because the surgeon will operate in flexion, midflexion, and extension surgical windows.

Instruments

MIS TKA must be performed with accurate instruments specially developed for the procedure. It is not possible to perform the operation with the traditional instruments developed for the open approach. The conventional instruments do not fit into the knee joint and do not allow visualization of the joint while the cuts and balancing are performed. The visual appearance is totally different and new. Surgeons must learn to interpret

a completely new image of the knee joint while continuing to apply the basic principles that they have learned. The instruments are a critical part of this new technology and are essential for its success. New instruments that are roughly half the size of traditional instruments have been developed to facilitate MIS TKA. (Further details about the specially developed instruments are available online at http://www.europe.stryker.com/.)

Pre-operative Planning

Pre-operative assessment must include a thorough physical examination and proper plain radiographic studies. At the physical examination, the Pre-operative deformity, range of motion, and laxity of the joint at different knee position should be documented. The Pre-operative radiographs should document deformity and malalignment, osteophytes, bone defects, and loose bodies. The Pre-operative posterior slope of the tibial cut should be measured on the conventional lateral radiographs at 30° of knee flexion, to plan this slope on surgical setting.[16]

Anesthesia Technique

Anesthesia in MIS TKA should provide adequate pain relief and muscle relaxation during the procedure and minimize post-operative pain. For post-operative pain control, the author's patients receive first a single sciatic nerve block and then a continuous femoral nerve block.[49,50] Regional techniques are performed on conscious, only slightly premedicated patients (5–10 µg of sufentanyl administered intravenously shortly before starting the procedure), using a neurostimulation device (Stimuplex HNS 11, Braun Melsungen AG, Melsungen, Germany) and stimulating needles.

The single-shot sciatic nerve block

The sciatic nerve is the largest nerve in the body, measuring about 2 cm in thickness in its proximal portion. At this location, it actually is composed of the sciatic nerve and the posterior cutaneous nerve of the thigh. This double nerve contains contributions from the lumbar nerve roots 4 and 5 and the sacral nerve roots 1, 2, and 3.

The single-shot sciatic nerve block is performed using the classical Labat approach with the patient in the lateral position, exposing the affected side (**Fig. 2**).[49] The needle (Polymedic UPC G23, 150 mm; Polymedic, TeMe Na, Carrieres sur Seine, France) is advanced toward the sciatic nerve until foot movements can be elicited at a threshold of 0.4 mA, 0.1 msec. A total of 15 to 20 mL ropivacaine 0.75% (Naropin®) is administered. This dose usually provides satisfactory analgesia for

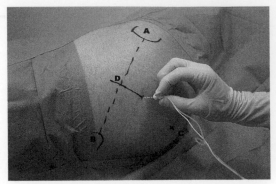

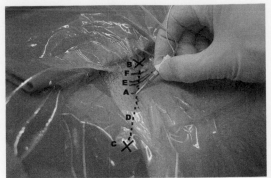

Fig. 2. The single sciatic nerve block is done following the technique of Labat:[49] The patient first is placed in the lateral position with the side to be blocked up. While the lower leg is kept straight, the thigh is flexed at the knee so that the ankle is brought over the knee of the other leg. The important bony landmarks to block the sciatic nerve via the two posterior approaches are the greater trochanter (A), the posterior superior iliac spine (B), and the ischial tuberosity (C). A line is drawn between the greater trochanter (A) and the posterior superior iliac spine (B). The line lies approximately over the upper border of the piriformis muscle. From the midpoint of this line (D) and at right angles to it, a second line is drawn passing over the buttock. The point of injection is 3 to 5 cm along this perpendicular line. It can be identified more precisely by drawing a third line between the greater trochanter and sacral hiatus; the point of injection is the intersection of this third line with the second, perpendicular line.

more than 24 hours. Alternatively, especially in immobile patients, the anterior[51] or lateral[52] approach for IB (sciatic block modified according to Meier) can be used.[53,54]

The continuous femoral nerve block

The femoral nerve receives contributions from the second, third, and fourth lumbar nerves. It is derived from the lumbar plexus and in fact lies within the same fascial envelope as the lumbar plexus. Therefore a single injection distally may be utilized to block most of the nerves originating in the lumbar plexus, because local anesthetic can pread proximally within this plane.

The femoral nerve block is performed with the patient in the supine position (**Fig. 3**). The catheter is placed using the classic paravascular Winnie approach.[50] The needle (Borgeat C 70T, Polymedic) is advanced until contractions of the quadriceps femoris muscle, at a threshold of 0.4 mA, 0.1 msec, indicate accurate positioning of the needle tip in the immediate proximity of the femoral nerve. After negative aspiration, 5–10 mL of NaCl 0.9% is injected. The needle is removed, and the catheter advanced 5 to 10 cm through

Fig. 3. The femoral nerve block is performed with the patient supine following the technique of Winnie.[50] The important bony landmarks for blocking the femoral nerve (A) are the pubic tubercle (B), the anterior superior iliac spine (C), the inguinal ligament (D), the lateral border of the femoral artery (E), and the femoral vein (F) at the inguinal crease. For the femoral nerve (A), the point of injection lies just below (distal to) the inguinal ligament (D). Palpate both the anterior superior iliac spine (C) and the pubic tubercle (B). The line between these two points overlies the inguinal ligament (D). It often is helpful to draw lines on the skin. The femoral artery (E) should lie at the midpoint of the inguinal ligament, and it is necessary to locate the artery by palpating the pulse at this point. The injection site is 1 cm lateral to lateral edge of the pulse of the femoral artery and 1 to 2 cm below (distal to) the line of the inguinal ligament.

the plastic cannula. After subcutaneous tunneling (5 cm) and application of a bacterial filter, 5–10 mL of lidocaine 1% is injected.

Because of the inconsistent blockade of the obturator nerve with the previously described blocks, the operation is performed with an additional lumbar spinal anesthesia (hyperbaric bupivacaine 0.5%, 2.5–3 mL) administered using a Reganesth Pencil Point G27 needle (Reganesth, Villingen, Germany) or general anesthesia (ie, propofol, remifentanil).

Immediately post-operatively, the femoral catheter is connected to a patient-controlled analgesia pump delivering ropivacaine 0.2%, usually set at a basic rate of 6 mL/h, with a 4-mL bolus function and a 30-minute lockout time. The setting then is adjusted according to the individual patient's pain scores and symptoms (particularly motor blockade) during daily ward rounds. The femoral catheter usually is left in place for 48 to 72 hours, depending on the individual patient's requirement.

Surgical Procedure

The patient is placed supine on a standard operating table. A tourniquet is applied after exsanguination of the limb, and standard skin preparation and draping are undertaken. Two fixed leg holders on the operating table allow flexion and extension of the lower limb for exposure. Flexing the knee exposes the posterior structures of the knee, and extending the knee exposes the anterior structures of the knee.

Navigation trackers pin position

The procedure is initiated by positioning one tracker on the distal femur and one tracker on the proximal tibia within the surgical access zone. These trackers are fixed rigidly to the bone so that their position in relation to the anatomically selected points remains constant, and any movement of the bone and its associated tracker position is recorded. The femoral tracker is fixed rigidly to the femur with the Ortholock, a femoral tracker fixing device (Stryker-Leibinger, Freiburg, Germany) with two bi-cortical predrilled pins (3 mm in diameter and 150 mm long) through stab wounds along the iliotibial tract 10 cm proximal to the patellar pole in an anterolateral to posteromedial direction. The tibial tracker is fixed with a special antirotational fixation pin through a small stab wound into the proximal tibia 15 cm distal to the tibial tuberosity. The information regarding the position of the trackers, the attached bone, and the instruments is analyzed by the computer, which determines the real-time position of the leg within a three-dimensional coordinate system. In the most recent modification of the system, only two trackers, one fixed to the distal femur and one fixed to the proximal tibia, are necessary.

Surgical approach

The author's preferred approach is the minimally invasive midvastus approach, with a length of approximately 8 cm in extension and 10 cm in flexion. The skin and underlying subcutaneous tissue are incised to expose the underlying retinaculum of the knee. At the superior end of the wound the fibers of the VMO are seen to insert into the medial aspect of the patella. A 2-cm stab wound is made in the VMO fibers at the edge of the patella in the 10 o'clock or 2 o'clock position, depending on the operative side. The incision then is continued along the medial side of the patella to the inferior aspect of the wound (see **Fig. 1**). With the leg in extension and two soft tissue retractors appropriately placed, the suprapatellar pouch is visible. The anterior capsule, a fine white fibrous layer, is dissected with Meztenbaum scissors and is divided longitudinally. The fat and synovial tissue over the anterior surface of the distal femur are removed, and any plical bands attaching the medial capsular layer to the medial

side of the femur are divided. The same process is accomplished on the lateral aspect. With the knee in extension, the patella is osteotomized freehand to a bone thickness of 12 mm for later resurfacing. This process allows further visualization of the lateral gutter (**Fig. 4**).

Through the distal medial arthrotomy wound, the anterior horn of the medial meniscus is excised. Care is taken to limit the excision of the fat pad beneath the patella tendon to avoid contracture of the patellar tendon. An interval is produced on the medial aspect releasing the anteromedial knee capsule/retinaculum from the anterior surface of the tibia and allowing visualization of the medial aspect of the knee. With the knee in mid-flexion/extension, a Langenbeck retractor is placed under the patellar tendon close to its insertion in the tibia. The surgeon now can visualize the anterolateral surface of the tibia, and the anterior horn of the lateral meniscus can be removed under direct vision.

Data analysis and bone resection

The digitizing pointer then is used to mark the key anatomic landmarks. The anatomic landmarks of the femur condyle must be prepared very precisely intraoperatively (**Figs. 5** and **6**).

After digitalization of the multiple landmarks, the surgeon can reproduce the correct joint kinematics with the Knee Navigation System (**Fig. 7**).

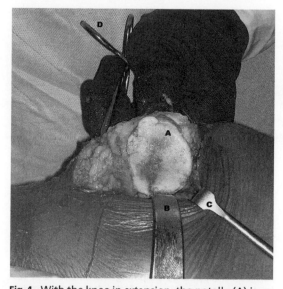

Fig. 4. With the knee in extension, the patella (A) is osteotomized freehand with the saw. The lateral femoral condyle is protected with a double femoral retractor (B), and the vastus medialis muscle is protected by a small Langenbeck retractor (C). Care must be taken not to injure the patellar and quadricepital tendons, which are held with two Backhaus clamps (D).

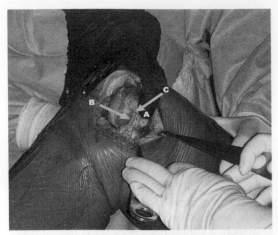

Fig. 5. Through the medial incision the surgeon prepares the medial epicondyle of the femur (A). To digitalize the medial epicondyle clearly with the pointer (B), the surgeon identifies the attachment of the superficial fibers of the medial collateral ligament attaching to the crescent-shaped prominence on the bony ridge of the medial epicondyle (C) and of the deep fibers of the medial collateral ligament in the sulcus.

After analyzing the kinematics curves and axis, bone cuts are performed using the information obtained from the navigation system. The author usually starts with the tibial cut. The proximal tibial

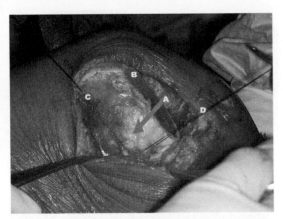

Fig. 6. During the initial anatomic landmark registration, the lateral epicondyle of the femur (A) can be palpated only approximately. After resection of the distal femur (see **Fig. 11**), (B), the lateral epicondyle can be remapped by palpating the smaller and less protuberant prominence of the lateral epicondyle (A), which corresponds to the attachment of the fibular collateral ligament of the knee (C). On the lateral surface of the lateral femoral condyle, the surgeon can visualize the origin of the popliteus muscle (D), anterior and inferior to the lateral epicondyle, which courses under the lateral collateral ligament and descend into the popliteus hiatus.

cut is made in one step, controlling the posterior slope, varus/valgus, and depth. The posterior slope of the tibial cut is aimed to match the original posterior slope of the tibial plateau.[16] The cutting guide with the resection plane probe is placed in the wound and the medial soft tissue envelope. Using the freehand technique, the surgeon adjusts the position of the probe according to the image and data shown on the computer. The guide is held using a tripod grip, and the visual movements of the guide can be monitored in real time on the screen (**Fig. 8**A, B).

Once the cutting guide is set in the final position, the block is secured into place with three pins, and the proximal tibial resection is performed with the saw blade (**Fig. 9**A). After the resected part of the tibia plateau is removed, the resection plane probe is used to verify the accuracy of the cut and to record the final cut on the screen (**Fig. 9**B).

The femoral distal cuts then are made as a two-step process, using the two femoral cutting blocks, the cutting guide, the femoral alignment guide, and the resection plane probe. The author begins with the distal femoral resection, which requires control of flexion/extension, varus/valgus, and depth of bone resection (**Fig. 10**).

After the distal femoral portion has been resected, the rotational landmarks of the femur are reviewed and, if necessary, remapped using the pointer. The rotational alignment subsequently is established with the femoral alignment guide and resection plane probe. The femoral component rotation is aimed to be $0°$ in relation to the special algorithm of surgical transepicondylar axis and the Whiteside line as provided by the computer software. With the computer-assisted navigation it possible to avoid an anterior femoral notching during the preparation of the distal femur and the femoral component can be aligned in the requested flexion (**Fig. 11**A–D).

Care is taken to release any flexion contracture, to remove all the posterior femoral osteophytes, and to align the femoral component in $1°$ of flexion, with the navigation system in the sagittal plane. The author then measures the femoral size with the femoral sizing guide, and finishes the preparation of the trochlea of the femur with trochlea resection guide. The femoral component then is inserted and, once it is seated correctly, the fixation lugholes are drilled (**Fig. 12**).

Subsequently, the tibial bone resection is finalized. The appropriately sized tibial baseplate is inserted, and the tibial component rotation is determined through self-adjustment by flexing and extending the knee with the trial femoral component implanted. The tibial component

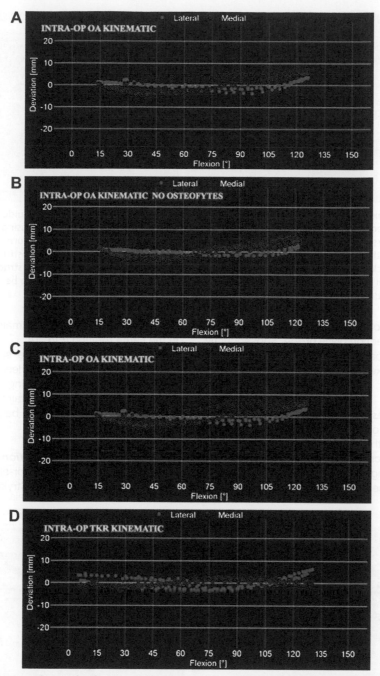

Fig. 7. (*A–D*) Progressive release of soft tissue. After the resection of the osteophytes, the surgeon can restore the correct joint kinematics with a progressive appropriate release of the soft tissue using initial kinematics quantified by the navigation technique to achieve parallel lengthening of the collateral ligaments through the entire range of motion.

rotation then is noted, and later the component is implanted with the desired rotation (**Fig. 13**).[55,56]

Trial component insertion

Before the trial components are inserted, the tibial and femoral bone cuts are verified with a small resection plane probe that is applied directly on the affected bone. Each bone cut performed is recorded and stored by the system and can be used for post-operative evaluation. After the tibial, femoral, and soft tissue preparation is complete and the trial components have been inserted, the

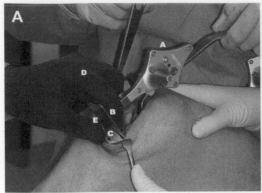
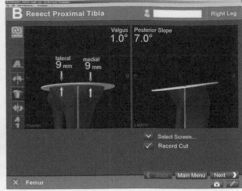

Fig. 8. (*A*) The proximal tibial resection requires the surgeon to position the MIS cutting guide in relation to the three axes of freedom controlling the varus/valgus, the depth, and the posterior slope, using a freehand technique. The universal tracker (A) is attached to the resection plane probe (B), which in turn is placed into the captured slot of the cutting guide (C). The surgeon holds the cutting guide/tracker construct using a "tripod grip" (D). The block is secured in place with three pins (E). (*B*) The cutting guide/tracker construct is now an active tool whose virtual position (ie, the varus/valgus angle, the slope angel and the depth) can be monitored on the computer navigation screen.

correct position of the trial components is checked with a small resection plane probe. Subsequently, the patella preparation is finished, and patellar tracking is checked with the trial implants in place.

Soft tissue assessment of trial components

After the insertion of the components, the limb alignment and the soft tissue balancing are assessed on the screen with the intraoperative kinematics by moving the limb from extension to deep flexion under neutral, varus, and valgus stress

through the heel of the foot, maintaining the limb in the same rotation (**Fig. 14**).

Using this information, the surgeon can plan any changes in the polyethylene insert and soft tissue release before repeating the assessment. In this way the surgeon obtains constant feedback during the process of balancing the knee (**Fig. 15**).

Definitive component Insertion

All patients receive a posterior-stabilized Scorpio knee total prosthesis (Stryker Howmedica

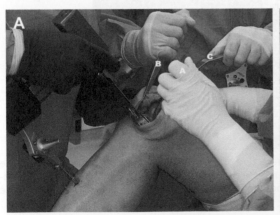
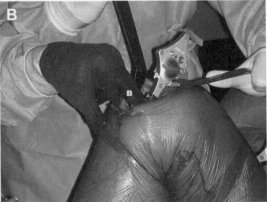

Fig. 9. (*A*) Proximal tibial resection with the saw blade. With the knee flexed, two retractors protect the soft tissue on the medial (A) and lateral side (B), and a giraffe retractor (C) is placed posteriorly to deliver the tibia lightly forward. Two retractors are necessary to protect important anatomic tissue: at the medial margin of the tibia plateau (A) to protect the medial collateral ligament and at the posterolateral corner of the tibia (B) to protect the popliteus tendon and the lateral genicular vessels. (*B*) After every bony resection, the universal tracker with the resection plane probe (A) can be placed flush on the cut surface to verify the accuracy of the cut (B). The surgeon can correct the cut by cutting freehand with the saw blade. Finally, the surgeon can record the tibial cut on the screen.

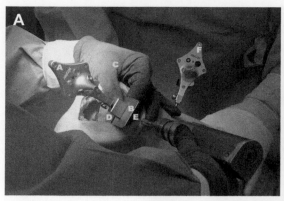
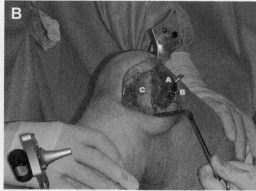
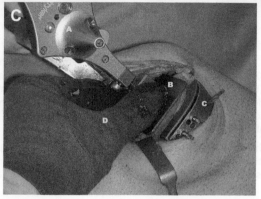

Fig. 10. (*A*) Distal femoral resection. The same cutting guide is used with the universal tracker (A) with the resection plane probe (B) placed in the captured slot (C). A similar freehand technique of cutting guide (D) placement is also used for the distal femoral resection. The block is pinned into place with three pins (E). The femoral tracker (F) is visible in this picture. (*B*) The cutting block (A) is fixed with three pins (B), and the surgeon uses a saw blade to effect the desired distal femoral resection (C). In this picture, the femoral and tibial trackers are also visable. (*C*) After the bony resection, the universal tracker (A) with the resection plane probe (B) can be used to verify the accuracy of the cut, to recorrect the resection if necessary, and finally to record the distal femoral cut on the screen. In the picture, the cutting block (C) is visible, and the freehand technique (D) of holding the universal tracker with the resection plane probe is demonstrated.

Osteonics, Freiburg, Germany). All femoral and tibial components are cemented with the Stryker Compact Vacuum Cement Mixing System. With the knee in deep flexion, two curved retractors are placed into the medial and lateral tibial plateau, and one retractor is placed posteriorly to deliver the tibia forward. The Scorpio tibial baseplate then is inserted into the keel cut and is cemented into position while its location is controlled with the resection plane probe (**Fig. 16**).

Any excess bone cement is removed under direct vision. In the same way, the Scorpio femoral component is cemented into the femur (**Fig. 17**), a trial polyethylene inlay is inserted, and thereafter the patellar component is embedded with cement (**Fig. 18**).

After the cement is fully polymerized, the tourniquet is released, and accurate hemostasis is performed. At this point it still is possible to assess the joint and soft tissue balance using trial polyethylene inlays of different sizes and to show the final kinematics analysis on screen, before the surgeon makes the final choice of insert size.

Closure

The joint is irrigated thoroughly, and a drain is inserted. The arthrotomy is closed with interrupted Vicryl 2-0 absorbable sutures with the knee at 90° of flexion. The subcutaneous layer is closed with Vicryl 2-0 sutures, and the skin is closed with Ethycrin 4-0 sutures (**Fig. 19**).

Subsequently, the final kinematics and outcome are documented, recorded, and compared with the initial kinematics data to assess the success of any correction (**Fig. 20**A, B). The data can be printed out and kept in the patient's record.

Postoperative Treatment

Peri- and post-operative pain treatment includes epidural anesthetic for 2 to 4 days and oral

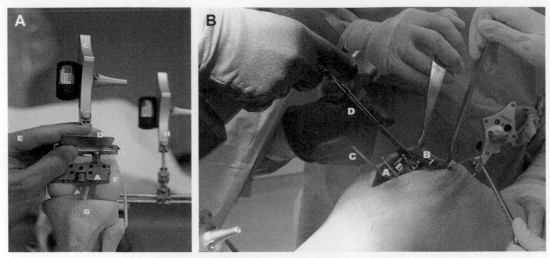

Fig. 11. (*A*) This picture shows on a model the adjustment of the femoral rotation with the base block (A), the anterior skim cutting guide (B), and the universal tracker (C) with the resection plane probe (D), which are placed with the freehand technique (E) into the desired rotation of the femoral component (F) and then pinned in place. The anterior skim cutting guide (B) is then raised flush with the anterior cortex of the distal femur avoiding dorsal notching of the distal femur cortex. The distal dorsal femoral cut can be performed with the saw blade. The proximal tibia (G) and the femoral tracker (H) are visible in the picture.

Fig. 11. (*B*) This picture shows the intra-operative view with the minimally invasive approach for the adjustment of the femoral component rotation. The femoral alignment guide with the base block (A) and the anterior skim cutting guide (B) have been secured with three pins (C). The distal dorsal femoral cut can be performed with the saw blade (D).

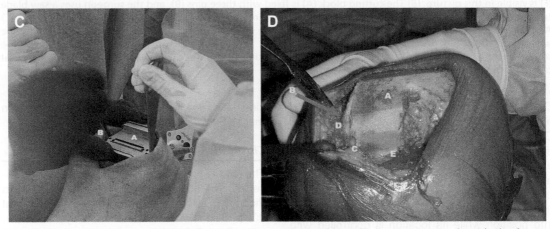

Fig. 11. (*C*) This picture shows the intra-operative view with the minimally invasive approach with the femoral resection guide in situs (A). After the distal dorsal femoral cut has been performed and the corrected femoral component rotation has been checked with the resection plane probe, the femoral component size can be selected. The appropriate size of the femoral resection guide (A) is chosen, placed onto the distal femoral cut surface, and secured with four pins (B, here with only one pin for this picture). The distal femoral cut can be finished with the saw blade.

Fig. 11. (*D*) This picture shows the intra-operative after performing all the distal femoral cuts. The resection level of each surface of the distal femur (A) can be measured with the resection plane probe and checked for accuracy. The thick red arrow (B) points to the lateral epicondyle. Two retractors are protecting the popliteus tendon (C), the lateral collateral ligament (D), and the soft tissue structures. The postero-lateral femur condyles (E) can now be cut with a curved osteotome, and the posterior capsule released and excised. The same step will be done for the medial femur condyle in the same way.

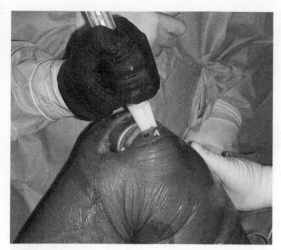

Fig. 12. Insertion of the femoral component. With the lateral and medial retractors still in place, the femoral implant is placed onto the distal femur (A) with the femoral impactor (B) to achieve correct positioning of the femoral component. This positioning can be verified again with the resection plane probe and visualized on the screen.

analgesics. Physical therapy is started as early as 5 to 6 hours post-operatively under the supervision of a physiotherapist (ie, continuous passive motion 3 times a day, early ambulation, walking exercises, active bending and extending exercises, active knee stretching exercises, walking up and down stairs, ergometer-bicycle riding, coordination exercises, rising from a seated position,

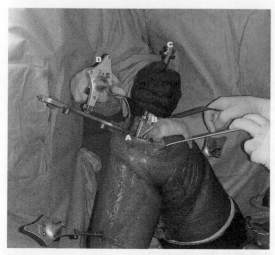

Fig. 13. Tibial rotation. The baseplate (A) is secured onto the tibial surface in the desired rotation. Then the preparation of the tibial keel is undertaken using the tibial punch tower (B) and tibial punches (C) under visual control on the screen with the universal tracker (D).

strengthening exercises, and other regimens). Patients are allowed to full weight bearing as tolerated. Patients are discharged from the hospital once they are able to flex the knee joint to 120°, perform an unassisted straight-leg raise, walk independently with or without crutches, rise from a chair to a standing position and sit from a standing position without support, and ascend and descend a full flight of stairs. All patients receive low molecular weight heparin for deep venous thrombosis prophylaxis for 6 weeks. Outpatient physical therapy is started after discharge. Patients are evaluated clinically and radiographically in the office at 6 weeks, 3 months, and 6 months.

CLINICAL EXPERIENCE WITH MINIMALLY INVASIVE COMPUTER-ASSISTED TOTAL KNEE ARTHROPLASTY

The author and his colleagues performed a comparative study in which 20 patients who had undergone conventional CN-TKA were compared with a directly matched group who had undergone MIS CN-TKA.[57]

Clinical Results

The two groups were matched according to gender, age, diagnosis, pre-operative deformity, etiology, range of motion, pre-operative Hospital for Special Surgery (HSS) knee score, Knee Society knee and function scores, major comorbidities, and duration of follow-up.[58,59] There were 11 women and 9 men in the conventional CN-TKA group and 12 women and 8 men in the MIS CN-TKA group. The mean pre-operative age was 67 years (range 37–87 years) for the conventional CN-TKA group and 68 years (range 48–76 years) for the MIS CN-TKA group. The mean pre-operative flexion was 120° (range 110°–130°) for the conventional CN-TKA group and 118° (range 110°–127°) for the MIS CN-TKA group. The mean pre-operative mechanical axis was 4.5° valgus (range 18° varus/16° valgus) for the conventional CN-TKA group and 4.7° valgus (range 16° varus/ 13° valgus) for the MIS CN-TKA group. No significant differences between the two groups were seen for age, gender, pre-operative mechanical axis, flexion, HSS knee score, functional knee score, and American Knee Society score. Inclusion and exclusion criteria and further demographic data are available on request from the author.[57] In the conventional CN-TKA group a standard medial parapatellar approach was used, whereas in the MIS CN-TKA group a midvastus approach was used.

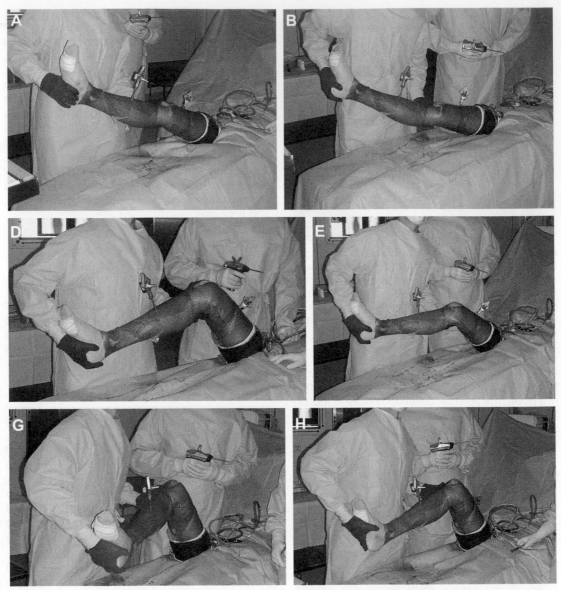

Fig. 14. The assessment of the joint kinematics with the computer-navigation: The kinematics of the knee can be assessed in a dynamic way moving the knee joint from maximal extension to deep flexion under no stress (Figures A, D, G), under manual varus stress (Figures B, E, H) and under manual valgus stress (Figures C, F, I) by maintaining the limb in the same rotation through the heel of the foot. The first line (Figures A-B-C) represents the knee joint position in 0° flexion/extension, the second line (Figures D-E-F) the knee joint position in 45° flexion/extension and the third line (Figures G-H-I) the knee joint position in 90° flexion/extension.

No difficulties in exposure and visualization were encountered in obese patients, patients with large knees, muscular male patients, or patients with more severe deformities. The author and his colleagues also have had no complications with the navigation system or reference pins. No complications (ie, fracture, revision, manipulation, deep infection, hematoma, clinically evident deep vein thrombosis, or major cardiopulmonary complication) occurred intraoperatively or postoperatively. There was no compromised implant fixation evident on follow-up. All patients recovered well after the operation.

The mean post-operative range of motion after the first 3 months was significantly higher in the MIS CN-TKA group (125°) than in the conventional CN-TKA group (118°) ($P = .037$). Six months after the operation, however, there was no statistically

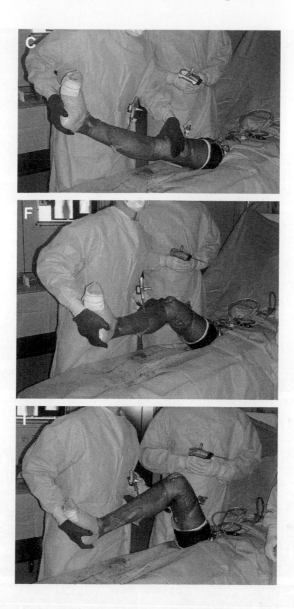

Fig. 14. (*continued*)

relevant difference between the two groups in range of motion (125° versus 122°). The HSS knee score improved in both groups to almost identical values during the first 6 months after the operation. The Knee Society clinical rating score (ie, the knee and function scores) also showed no significant difference between the groups during the first 6 months after surgery. The author and his colleagues found no statistically significant differences between the MIS CN-TKA group and the conventional CN-TKA group in operating time and blood loss.

Radiographic Results

All patients received full-length standing antero-posterior radiographs pre-operatively and 6 weeks postoperatively. Full-length full-weight-bearing standing anteroposterior radiographs were performed with the automated Philips Multidiagnost 3 (Philips Medical Systems, DMC GmbH, Hamburg, Deutschland). Pre- and post-operative mechanical axes (ie, the coronal mechanical axis of the limb, the hip-knee angle) were determined from radiographs. A mechanical axis of more than 3° varus/valgus was determined as an outlier, as defined previously.[17,18] Conventional radiographic assessment involved short-leg-length weight-bearing anteroposterior radiographs, as well as nonrotated short-leg-length lateral radiographs at 30° of knee flexion and patella axial radiographs pre-operatively and 6 months after the operation. The alignment of the prosthetic

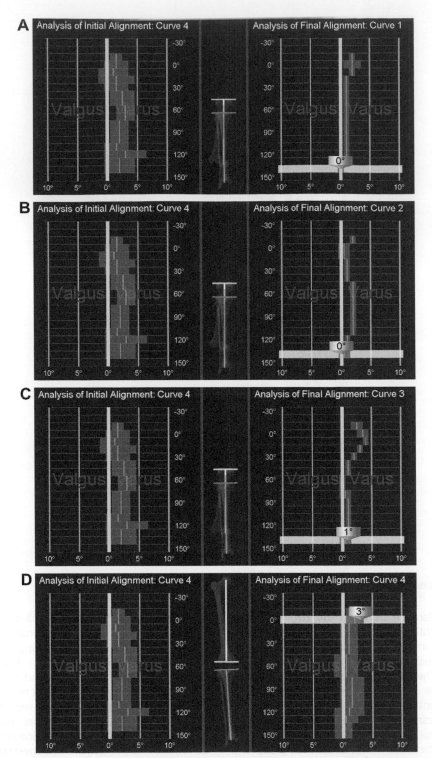

Fig. 15. The range of motion, the alignment of the limb, and the stability of the medial and lateral joint space can be verified, recorded and compared to the initial kinematics data on the screen under no stress (A), under manual varus stress (B), and under manual valgus stress (C). It still is possible at this stage to assess the complete joint stability and soft tissue balance under maximal varus and valgus stress by using different sizes of polyethylene trials and the final kinematic analysis screen (D) prior to inserting the definitive insert size.

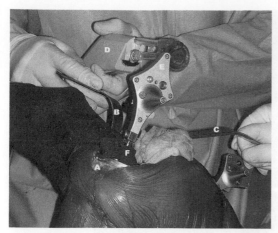

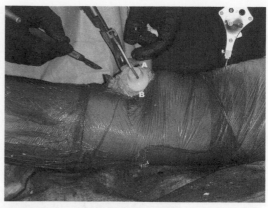

Fig. 18. The patellar component (A) is inserted with cement (B), which can be removed with a knife under good visualization.

Fig. 16. Definitive insertion of the tibial baseplate component (A). With the knee flexed, two retractors are used to protect the soft tissues on the medial and lateral aspect (B). A giraffe retractor (C) is placed posteriorly to deliver the tibia lightly forward. After the tibial surface is cleaned with the pulsating lavage device (D), the tibial baseplate (A) is inserted into the keel cut and cemented down into the desired position, which is checked with the universal tracker (E) and the resection plane probe (F).

components was evaluated on the short-leg-length standard radiographs. Radiographic parameters including the coronal femoral component angle, the sagittal femoral component angle, the coronal tibial component angle, and the sagittal tibial component angle (ie, tibial slope

angle) were evaluated to assess the correct positioning of the femoral and tibial components.[60] The coronal alignment of the femoral component was measured in relation to the anatomic femoral axis (ideal value 96°) and of the tibial component in relation to the anatomic tibial axis (ideal value 90°) (**Fig. 21**). To determine the sagittal angle of the femoral and tibial components respectively, a perpendicular line drawn from the midline of the femoral tibial components was compared with the midline of the distal segment of the femur and of the proximal segment of the tibia using the Knee Society score reference lines.[61] Although there is little consensus about the ideal reference for measuring the slope of the tibia on the lateral radiograph, the author and his colleagues used the technique described by Catani and colleagues[16] and Yoo and colleagues[62] measuring the slope of the tibial component on conventional short-length sagittal-view radiographs with

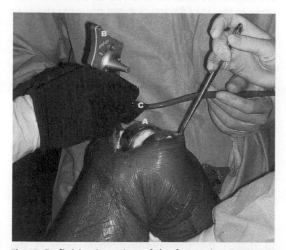

Fig. 17. Definitive insertion of the femoral component. After the femoral surface is cleaned with a pulsating lavage device, the femoral component (A) is inserted and cemented in the desired position, which is checked with the universal tracker (B) and the resection plane probe (C). When the component is in the desired position, any excess cement can be removed.

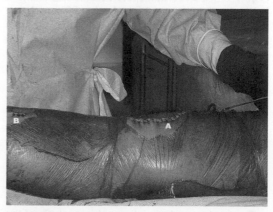

Fig. 19. The wound (A) is closed, and the pins, including the trackers, are removed. (B) marks the tibial wound.

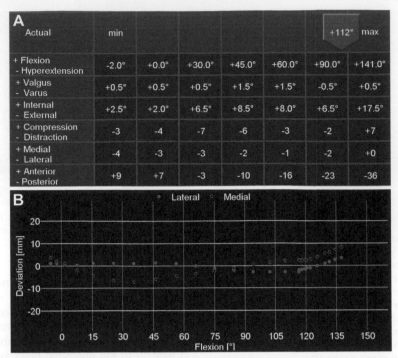

Fig. 20. The final kinematics and outcome are documented on the screen as a value (A) and as a curve (B).

reference to the proximal anatomic axis. The pre- and post-operative sagittal tibial component angle (ie, tibial slope angle) was compared on conventional short-length lateral radiographs in 30° of knee flexion.

The radiographic coronal mechanical axis of the limb (ie, the hip-knee angle) improved to normal values in both groups (0.5° in the conventional CN-TKA group and 0.7° in the MIS CN-TKA group). There were no alignment outliers in the mechanical axis in either group postoperatively (Fig. 21). With regard to the accuracy of the coronal alignment of the femoral component (ideal value 96° in relation to the anatomic femoral axis), the author and his colleagues found a correct implantation of the femoral component in all cases, with no statistically significant differences between the conventional CN-TKA group (mean value 96.2°) and MIS CN-TKA group (mean value 95.2°) (see Fig. 21). They found the same accuracy for the implantation of the tibial component in the coronal alignment (ideal value 90° in relation to the anatomic and mechanical tibial axes), with no statistically significant differences between the conventional CN-TKA group (mean value 91.3°) and the MIS CN-TKA group (mean value 91.4°) (Fig. 21).

The post-operative radiographic analysis of the sagittal alignment of the femoral component in relation to the anatomic femoral axis revealed slightly greater flexion of the femoral components in both groups in comparison with pre-operative planning (mean value 6.9° in the conventional CN-TKA group versus 7.8° in the MIS CN-TKA group) (Fig. 22). The intraoperative alignment of the sagittal femoral cut showed an accurate value close to the 1° of flexion planned pre-operatively in both the conventional CN-TKA group (mean value 0.58°, SD 0.44°, range 0.0°–1.5°) and the MIS CN-TKA group (mean value 1.03°, SD 0.40°, range 0.5°–2.0°). This difference might be explained by the use of different methods to determine the sagittal femoral components angle intraoperatively and postoperatively. The intraoperative measurements of femoral bone resection in the sagittal plane were assessed with the navigation system, which measures this angle in relation to the mechanical axis, whereas the post-operative measurements were performed with a short-leg lateral radiograph at 30° of knee flexion, which defines this angle in relation to the anatomic axis of the femur. The tibial slope was reconstructed to match the pre-operative value both in the conventional CN-TKA group (mean value 1.6°) and in the MIS CN-TKA group (mean value 1.4°) (Fig. 22).

All patients also received standardized CT scans of both knees 6 weeks postoperatively to evaluate rotational alignment of the components.[63]

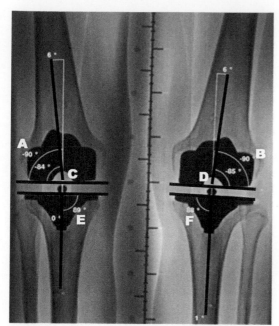

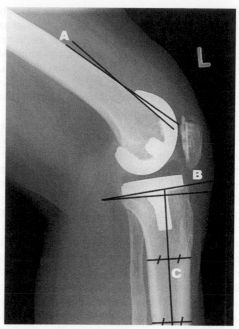

Fig. 21. The postoperative mechanical axes (A and B angles) (ie, the coronal mechanical axis of the limb) (*white line*) after a bilateral MIS CN TKA with straight axes on both sides. The coronal alignment of the femoral component is measured in relation to the anatomic femoral axis (*black line in the femur canal;* ideal value 96°) and of the tibial component in relation to the anatomic tibial axis (*black line in the tibial canal;* ideal value 90°). The coronal alignments of the femoral (angles C and D) and tibial components (angles E and F) are correct at both sides as well.

Fig. 22. Analyses of the sagittal alignment on postoperative short-leg-length lateral radiograph at 30° of knee flexion: the sagittal femoral component angle (angle A) and the sagittal tibial component angle (angle B) (ie, the tibial slope). The slope of the tibial component (B angle) is measured with reference to the proximal anatomic axis (C).

Multislice CT scans of the knees in 5-mm slice thickness and 2-mm slice distance were obtained using a GE Lightspeed multislice scanner (GE Medical Systems, (Schweiz) AG, Glattbrugg, Switzerland). The analysis of the post-operative CT scans revealed a statistically significant reconstruction of the desired rotational alignment of the femoral component parallel to the transepicondylar axis in both the conventional CN-TKA group (mean value 0.7°) and the MIS CN-TKA group (mean value 1.3°) ($P = .018$). The author and his colleagues were not able to document any outliers in terms of rotational alignment of the femoral prosthesis.

DISCUSSION

Malposition of TKA affects implant fixation and leads to an increased risk of loosening and instability and to decreased survival of the prosthesis. Computer-assisted navigation systems have been designed to increase the precision of TKA implantation. Computer-assisted TKA implantation allows the surgeon to reproduce the

mechanical axes measured on full-length standing radiographs of the lower limb and reduces the number of outliers in the alignment of the limb compared with traditional mechanical instrumented TKA.[9,23–27,29–31] Furthermore, although analysis of alignment and component orientation after computer-navigated and conventional implantation shows contradictory results, two recent meta-analyses of alignment outcome for computer-assisted versus conventional TKA indicate significant improvement in component orientation and mechanical axis when computer-assisted navigation is used.[64,65]

Our comparative study demonstrated that it is possible, by using a computer-assisted navigation system, to achieve straight mechanical axes using either a conventional or a minimally invasive approach. No outliers were found in either group. Furthermore, the intraoperative alignment of the femoral and tibial bone resection was accurate in all three planes in both the conventional CN-TKA and the MIS CN-TKA groups. Similar intraoperative results have been published, and our results showed the same accuracy using the navigation system the intraoperative bone resections as reported in the previous studies.[9,24–26,28]

The limits of these meta-analyses warrant further discussion, however, because the mechanical axis may be a parameter too simple to use as an indicator of limb alignment and better long-term outcomes. Accurate angles of the individual components in the coronal and sagittal plane, correct rotation, and proper ligament and soft tissue balancing contribute to the success of knee replacement surgery. Various studies have compared component orientation performed with computer-assisted systems versus traditional implantation. All these studies, however, have investigated TKA implanted using conventional approaches. Most authors showed that the coronal alignment (ie, the varus/valgus alignment) of the femoral component was improved with the use of computer navigation.[9,19,24-26,60,66-69] Only few studies did not report an improvement in component alignment when computer navigation was used.[70,71] Even though the senior authors in these studies have more experience with conventional TKA than with navigated TKA, there were fewer outliers in the navigation group. We were also able to demonstrate that, using a commercially available computer-assisted navigation system, it is possible to implant the femoral and tibial components in the desired coronal planes with either the conventional approach and with a minimally invasive approach. The post-operative radiographic analyses of the coronal alignment of the femoral and tibial components showed reliable results in both groups, without any outliers in either group.

Sagittal alignment of the femoral component can be improved with the use of navigation in conventional approaches.[9,19,24,25,30,66,67,69] We were able to implant the femoral and tibial components in the desired sagittal plane in MIS CN-TKA as well as in conventional CN-TKA.

The influence of navigation on the alignment of the tibial component remains unclear. Several authors confirmed that the coronal alignment of the tibial component (ie, the varus/valgus alignment) is improved with the use of navigation.[9,24,69] Other authors, however, did not find an improvement in the coronal alignment of the tibial component.[19,30,62,63] We found the same accuracy for the implantation of the tibial component in the coronal plane the conventional approach and in the minimally invasive approach. Furthermore, we showed that the sagittal-tibial component angle (ie, the tibial slope angle) can be reconstructed accurately and reproducibly to match the original value of the tibial plateau in both computer-assisted approaches. Although some studies did not find that the alignment in the sagittal plane of the tibial component was improved with navigation, our results confirmed, as has been reported by other authors, that the surgeon can use computer-assisted navigation as a practical means to restore the tibial slope accurately during MIS CN TKA.[19,24,25,28,30,67,72-74]

Debate still exists about whether a navigation system improves the rotational alignment of the femoral component.[75] Several reference axes have been proposed to establish proper rotational alignment of the femoral components.[72] Of these axes, the transepicondylar axis approximates the flexion-extension axis of the knee. Furthermore, although there is no consensus about the best landmarks to gauge femoral rotation, alignment according to the surgical epicondylar axis seems to come closest to allowing physiologic biomechanics.[7,8,10,76] Debate continues about how accurately and easily the transepicondylar axis can be located intraoperatively. In a cadaver study, Siston and colleagues[72] found high variability in the rotational alignment of the femoral component. This variability may be explained by the surgeon's greater or lesser ability to identify intraoperatively the medial epicondyle with its bone ridge and sulcus and the attachment of the deep and superficial fibers of the medial ligament (see **Fig. 5**), by the learning curve for the surgeon associated with the use of navigation, and by the skills of the individual surgeon. Stöckl and colleagues[25] reported the same accuracy in finding the proper femoral rotational alignment with a conventional approach as with the Stryker navigation system. The algorithm used by the Stryker Knee Navigation Software to establish the proper femoral rotational alignment by averaging the angle subtended by the Whiteside line and the transepicondylar axis makes it possible for the surgeon to improve the accuracy of the femoral rotational alignment without unduly increasing the operative time. The analysis of our post-operative rotational alignment of the femoral component by CT scans revealed a statistically significant reconstruction of the desired rotational alignment of the prosthesis parallel to the transepicondylar axis in both the conventional and the minimally invasive computer-assisted navigated approaches. We found no outliers of the femoral rotational alignment in either group. These results are in agreement with other studies using standard approaches, computer-assisted navigation, and an improved CT protocol.[24,25,77] Accuracy in adjusting the rotational alignment of the femoral component is a prerequisite to avoid malfunctioning TKAs. Even small abnormalities of the rotational alignment of the components have a considerable influence on patellar tracking, on stability, and on the overall biomechanics of the joint. To the author's knowledge, this study is the first comparative study using a CT technique and a minimally invasive approach that shows it is possible to adjust the rotational alignment of the femoral component accurately and reproducibly by using a computer-assisted navigation in both conventional and minimally invasive approaches.

Although it has been reported that the rotational mismatch between the femoral and tibial components is decreased with navigation, controversy still exists as to whether navigation systems improve the rotational alignment of the tibial component in the axial plane.[24,78] We used the technique describe by Dalury[55] and Eckhoff and colleagues[56] in which the orientation of the tibial tray was determined by allowing it to float into position with respect to the femoral component while the knee was placed through a full arc of motion and were able to document an accurate alignment of the tibial component in the CT scan. We believe, however, that a navigation system that relies only on digitization of landmarks to establish the rotational alignment of the tibial component is not sufficiently reliable. Therefore further research is necessary.

Component malpositioning is not the only cause of long-term TKA failure. Instability, often representing a failure to correct the soft tissue and to balance the flexion and extension gaps at the time of the index arthroplasty, can lead to implant failure. In some studies, 30% to 35% of revision TKAs were caused by an uncorrected joint stability.[20–22] Stability of the knee involves ligaments that behave differently on the medial and lateral aspects. Medial–lateral instability is the most common type of instability and may result from incompetent collateral ligaments, incomplete correction of a pre-operative deformity, incorrect bone cuts, or incorrect restoration of the original joint line. A stable knee joint maintains an appropriate minimum contact force between the articulating surfaces throughout the functional range of motion. Thus, a TKA is stable when, moving through its range of motion, it can undertake the required functional loads without pain, maintaining contact on nonperipheral located regions, and produce a joint contact force of normal intensity on the polyethylene insert. Any factors causing an abnormal joint contact force and/or an abnormal eccentric position of joint contact force might lead to polyethylene and component loosening. The TKA stability and function are related directly to the interplay among the implant component alignment, articular surface geometry (flat or congruent polyethylene insert), cruciate-retaining or cruciate-substituting prosthesis design, soft tissue balancing, and muscle action. Of these factors, implant component alignment, joint-line

restoration, and soft tissue balancing can be and should be assessed and restored by the surgeon during the surgery. The joint-line height both at the femur and tibia usually is calculated using measurements on pre- and post-operative radiographs and standard anatomic indices. The Knee Navigation System allows the surgeon to measure and restore the femoral joint height and the tibial joint line (**Fig. 23** A–C).[79]

To avoid incorrect location of the joint line, the surgeon can measure the tibial and femoral joint-line heights intraoperatively with the Knee Navigation System. The surgeon also can measure the variance of this line: the tibial joint-line variation is the difference between pre-operative and post-operative tibial heights; therefore a negative value indicates tibial elevation. A similar calculation can be performed on the femoral side.[79] These measurements, however, are affected by soft tissue release, which is difficult to quantify intraoperatively. Furthermore, an established concept has been the preparation of a rectangular joint gap in TKA. With a posterior-stabilized TKA, flexion and extension gaps can differ. A rectangular joint gap has been regarded as an important goal for achieving good joint function. The lateral tibiofemoral joint is physiologically lax, however, and as consequence the flexion gap may not be rectangular. In a cadaveric study on normal, non-arthritic knee joints, Van Damme and colleagues[80] reported greater lateral than medial laxity in full extension and increased lateral laxity from $0°$ to $90°$ flexion. Because of technical difficulties, few data are available on the physiologic laxity of the joint. Such analysis can be performed only if the flexed knee is imaged three-dimensionally both in neutral position and under a varus/valgus stress. Developments in MRI now allow the living knee to be imaged in a variety of positions and flexion angles. Tokuhara and colleagues[81] analyzed quantitatively the stability of the medial and lateral tibiofemoral joint for normal knees in open MRI. Their results indicate that the flexion gap in a normal knee is not rectangular and that the lateral joint gap is significantly lax. Recent biomechanical studies have shown further that flexion of the knee is associated with a significant medial-pivot internal rotation of the tibia.[82–85] Thus, in rotation the medial condyle is immobile, and the lateral condyle is mobile on the tibial surface. Since 1977, several studies using optical encoders, pressure-sensitive film, fluoroscopy, or a knee analysis system have investigated the relationship between soft tissue release and the resulting changes in the tibiofemoral gaps in TKA.[86–89] Most of these methods are difficult to use in routine TKA practice because of ergonomy, cost,

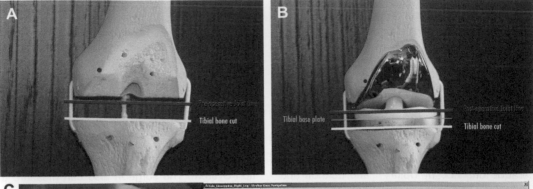

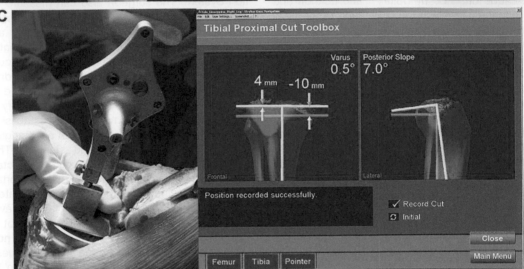

Fig. 23. Models showing measurement of the tibial joint line. (*A*) The height of the pre-operative tibial joint line (*red line*) is measured by digitalizing the deepest points on the two tibial condyles with the Knee Navigation System. The yellow line indicates the tibial bone cut. (*B*) The height of the postoperative tibial joint-line height (*red line*) is calculated by measuring the height of the tibial base plate with the resection plane probe and the thickness of the polyethylene. (*C*) Intraoperatively, the surgeon can measure the tibial joint line with the universal tracker with the resection plane probe (*left*). The corresponding medial and lateral heights are stored on the persona computer screen (*right*).

or safety. Computer-assisted surgical technology enables surgeons to measure and assess knee behavior during surgery, allowing real-time monitoring of the knee's behavior from extension to flexion and soft tissue balance. In a previous study, we measured the mechanical axis and the varus/valgus stability of the joint at different time points using the computer-assisted knee navigation, and we documented a similar increased lateral joint laxity before and after implantation of the components at 45° and 90° of knee flexion.[90] Therefore, knee navigation enables the surgeon to monitor and to quantify objectively what the surgeon used to feel and estimate in the past: the kinematics and stability of the TKA through the full range of motion pre-, intra- and postoperatively. Leaving the knee too lax after TKA

theoretically may lead to tibiofemoral instability, and excessive tightness may cause stiffness. The assessment of laxity is a new step in using the computer intraoperatively for balancing soft tissue safely. Unlike TKA alignment, however, no data are available to define a well-balanced knee intra- and/or postoperatively. As ideal laxity for TKA, we suggested a varus/valgus laxity of an approximately total joint-line opening between 1.5° to 2° to be achieved over the whole range of motion.[90] These findings serve as a benchmark for future measurements of soft tissue laxity, and these proposed values should be validated by additional work. The computer will help correlate the collected data and clinical outcomes more objectively than in the past and enable the setting of more accurate limits for soft tissue management.

Recently, various authors have reported superior clinical results and decreased cost using MIS techniques for TKA.[35,37,40,41] The conventional surgical approaches and instrumented techniques seem to cause much more soft tissue damage, leading to a very long recovery period. Although the length of the skin incision is shorter in the MIS approach, MIS knee surgery should not be defined by the size of the skin incision but rather by the method of soft tissue handling once the skin is incised. We believe that minimal trauma of the soft tissue and bone results in better post-operative function and accelerated rehabilitation. In our study, we were able to demonstrate that MIS CN-TKA can achieve these objectives. Although we could not find any statistical differences 6 months after the index operation, patients in the MIS CN-TKA group improved their range of motion faster than those in the conventional CN-TAK group. This difference was only significant 3 months postoperatively, however. These results are consistent with the experience of other studies on minimally invasive surgery.[31,41,91–93] Furthermore, there was no difference between the two groups in operation time or blood loss as measured by post-operative change in hemoglobin. With the minimally invasive approach, patients were mobilized more aggressively, reaching full weight bearing and leaving the hospital earlier. We also observed no significant differences between the conventional CN-TKA and MIS CN-TKA groups in HSS and Knee Society scores after 6 months. These clinical scores, however, are not ideal for the evaluation of patient satisfaction soon after a computer-navigated TKA with a conventional or MIS approach.[94] It would have been more appropriate to use patients' self-reported measures of outcome, such as the Western Ontario and McMaster Universities Index of Osteoarthritis and the Short Form-36 scoring systems.[43] In addition, a prospective, randomized, controlled study demonstrated a positive correlation between accurate mechanical alignment after TKA and functional and quality-of-life outcomes.[43] At all post-operative follow-up intervals from 6 weeks to 12 months, the total Knee Society score was significantly better in patients who had a mechanical axis within 3° of neutral than in those who had a mechanical axis greater than 3°. Moreover, the Short Form-12 (SF-12) physical scores at all intervals from 3 months on were significantly better for patients who had a mechanical axis within 3° of neutral, and at 12 months these patients demonstrated better SF-12 mental scores as well. Additionally, TKA with good alignment can lead to better function with quicker rehabilitation and earlier hospital discharge.[44] Therefore, the use of computer-assisted navigation leads not only to reproducible accuracy of implant positioning in all three planes but also to better functional outcomes with quicker rehabilitation and earlier hospital discharge because of the advantages of minimally invasive techniques.

POTENTIAL PITFALLS OF MINIMALLY INVASIVE COMPUTER-ASSISTED TOTAL KNEE ARTHROPLASTY

The primary risk of computer-assisted navigation is for the surgeon to lose perspective regarding the value of the system. The system is very sophisticated and, if used correctly, will improve accuracy. The system enhances the surgeon's perspective but should never replace it.

MIS CN-TKA is a more challenging procedure than a standard TKA. Complications may be reduced, but surgical risks to avoid include

- Excessive traction to the skin with skin breakdown
- Malfunctioning of the navigation system (ie, dirty reflectors, camera or rounding errors) or of the reference pin (ie, intraoperatively loosening of the pin and consequent inaccuracies in reference reading)
- Stretching against the quadriceps mechanism, which can cause intrinsic damage to or shredding of the muscle
- Inappropriate patella bone resection with the risk of a post-operative fracture or patella overstuffing
- Inaccurate identification of the anatomic landmarks at surgery
- Avulsion of the patellae tendon or injury to the patella by excessive traction on the patella
- Inappropriate bone cut caused by decreased visualization
- Inappropriate osteophytes/cement removal caused by decreased visualization
- Femoral and tibia mal rotation, malalignment, and malpositioning
- Difficult tibial keel preparation with risk of damaging the lateral femoral condyle
- Inadequate cement pressurization and implantation

Although excellent results may be achieved with computer-assisted navigation, certain factors still are cause for concern intraoperatively. If the patient has severe osteopenia, the pins placed in the bones to hold the trackers may become loose, making all further measurements inaccurate. Therefore, the surgeon must be very careful when handling pins and trackers. Likewise, because only the cutting guides are navigated, the surgeons may make less-than-optimal bone resections by bending the saw blade, especially when attempting to cut through sclerotic areas of bone. Also, differences in cement thickness may lead to malalignment, even though the bone resection was accurate. These latter two problems, which can occur with conventional instrumentation as well, can be obviated with the computed-assisted navigation only by using the verification plate of the Knee Navigation System, which allows the surgeon to check every cutting procedure during the operation and to verify the correct level of the joint line.

ADVANTAGES OF COMPUTER-ASSISTED MINIMALLY INVASIVE TOTAL KNEE ARTHROPLASTY

The use of computer-assisted navigation leads to reproducible accuracy of implant positioning in all three planes in both conventional and minimally invasive approaches. In contrast to even the most elaborate mechanical instrumentation system, which relies on visual inspection to confirm the accuracy of the alignment and stability of the TKA, computer-assisted navigation allows the surgeon to verify every operative cut by using the resection plane probe, which allows three-dimensional control of the cut planes on the screen, of the position of trial components, and finally of the position of the implants. In addition, computer-assisted technology assists the surgeon in reliably measuring the kinematics of TKA alignment and the stability of the TKA on a screen. Furthermore, surgeons have the opportunity to improve their surgical performance with a direct intraoperative documentation of the alignment and orientation of instruments, trial components, and implants. These advantages improve the accuracy of every single cut. Furthermore, the computer-assisted navigation allows the surgeon to verify the final alignment of the implants after component implantation and before the cement hardens, an ability the author believes is important to avoid considerable error in alignment. The conventional technique is limited by the dependence on extramedullary alignment guides or intramedullary rods. Correct positioning of the components, however, may only be a co-factor, together with instability and soft tissue trauma with the minimally invasive approach, leading to suboptimal implant loading with early loosening and increased wear. The use of computer-assisted navigation alone will not empower the surgeon to implant a TKA accurately and reproducibly, especially if the minimally invasive technique is used. Technical expertise in the conventional TKA and the surgeon's

skill and familiarity with the instruments also are necessary to obtain good results.

ACKNOWLEDGMENTS

The author acknowledges the work of Drs. M. Brouwer, F. Tichler, and M. Stephan, chairmen of the Spital Oberengadin Anesthesiology Department, who have contributed to the anesthesiology section of this article. He thanks Prof. Fabio Catani, Dr. Andrea Ensini, and their collaborators of the Istituti Ortopedici Rizzoli of Bologna, Italy, for their great personal commitment, help with the statistical analysis, and editorial review. He acknowledges the cooperation and support of the operating room personnel at the Spital Oberengadin, and the ongoing supervision of the Swiss Stryker Company.

REFERENCES

1. Callaghan JJ, O'Rourke MR, Iossi MF, et al. Cemented rotating-platform total knee replacement. A concise follow-up at a minimum of fifteen years. J Bone Joint Surg Am 2005;87:1995–8.
2. Gill GS, Joshi AB. Long-term results of kinematic condylar knee replacement: an analysis of 404 knees. J Bone Joint Surg Br 2001;83:335–58.
3. Pavone V, Boettner F, Fickert S, et al. Total condylar knee arthroplasty: a long term follow-up. Clin Orthop Relat Res 2001;388:18–25.
4. Ritter MA, Berend ME, Meding JB, et al. Long-term follow-up of anatomic graduated components posterior cruciate-retaining total knee replacement. Clin Orthop Relat Res 2001;388:51–7.
5. Rodrigues JA, Bhende H, Ranawat CS. Total condylar knee replacement: a 20-year follow-up study. Clin Orthop Relat Res 2001;388:10–7.
6. Insall JN, Binazzi R, Soudry M, et al. Total knee arthroplasty. Clin Orthop Relat Res 1985;192:13–22.
7. Insall JN, Scuderi GR, Komistek RD, et al. Correlation between condylar lift-off and femoral component alignment. Clin Orthop Relat Res 2002;403:143–52.
8. Barrack RL, Schrader T, Bertot AJ, et al. Component rotation and anterior knee pain after total knee arthroplasty. Clin Orthop Relat Res 2001;392:46–55.
9. Sparmann M, Wolke B, Czupalla H, et al. Positioning of total knee arthroplasty with and without navigation support. J Bone Joint Surg Br 2003;85:830–5.
10. Miller MC, Berger RA, Petrella AJ, et al. Optimizing femoral component rotation in total knee arthroplasty. Clin Orthop Relat Res 2001;392:38–45.
11. Nagamine R, White SE, McCarthy DS, et al. Effect of rotational malposition of the femoral component on knee stability kinematics after total knee arthroplasty. J Arthroplasty 1995;10:265–70.

12. Romero J, Duronio JF, Sohrabi A, et al. Varus and valgus flexion laxity of total knee alignment methods in loaded cadaveric knees. Clin Orthop Relat Res 2002;394:243–53.

13. Figgie HE, Goldberg VM, Heiple KG, et al. The influence of tibial-patellofemoral location on function of the knee in patients with posterior stabilized condylar knee prosthesis. J Bone Joint Surg Am 1986;68:1035–40.

14. Piazza SJ, Delp SL, Stulberg SD, et al. Posterior tilting of the tibial component decreases femoral rollback in posterior-substituting knee replacement: a computer simulation study. J Orthop Res 1998; 16:264–70.

15. Ritter MA, Faris PM, Keating EM, et al. Postoperative alignment of total knee replacement. Its effect on survival. Clin Orthop Relat Res 1994;299:153–6.

16. Catani F, Leardini A, Ensini A, et al. The stability of cemented tibial component of total knee arthroplasty: posterior cruciate-retaining versus posterior-stabilized design. J Arthroplasty 2004;19(6):775–82.

17. Jeffery RS, Morris RW, Denham RA. Coronal alignment after total knee replacement. J Bone Joint Surg Br 1991;73:709–14.

18. Rand JA, Coventry MB. Ten-year evaluation of geometric total knee arthroplasty. Clin Orthop Relat Res 1988;232:168–73.

19. Matziolis G, Krocher D, Weiss U, et al. A prospective, randomized study of computer-assisted and conventional total knee arthroplasty. J Bone Joint Surg Am 2007;89:236–43.

20. Lotke PA, Ecker ML. Influence of positioning of prosthesis in total knee replacement. J Bone Joint Surg Am 1977;59:77–9.

21. Nabeyama R, Matsuda S, Miura H, et al. The accuracy of image-guided knee replacement based on computed tomography. J Bone Joint Surg Br 2004; 86:366–71.

22. Sharkey PF, Hozack WJ, Rothman RH, et al. Insall Award paper: why are total knee arthroplasties failing today? Clin Orthop Relat Res 2002;404:7–13.

23. Stulberg S, Loan P, Sarin V. Computer-assisted navigation in total knee replacement: results of an initial experience in thirty-five patients. J Bone Joint Surg Am 2002;84:90–8.

24. Chauhan SK, Scott RG, Breidahl W, et al. Computer-assisted knee arthroplasty versus a conventional jig-based technique. A randomized, prospective trial. J Bone Joint Surg Br 2004;86(3):372–7.

25. Stöckl B, Nogler M, Rosiek R, et al. Navigation improved accuracy of rotational alignment in total knee arthroplasty. Clin Orthop Relat Res 2004;426: 180–6.

26. Bäthis H, Perlick L, Tingart M, et al. Alignment in total knee arthroplasty: a comparison of computer-assisted surgery with conventional technique. J Bone Joint Surg Br 2004;86:682–7.

27. Martin A, Wohlgenannt O, Prenn M, et al. Imageless navigation for TKA increased implant accuracy. Clin Orthop Relat Res 2007;460:178–84.

28. Ensini A, Catani F, Leardini A, et al. Alignments and clinical results in conventional and navigated total knee arthroplasty. Clin Orthop Relat Res 2007;457: 156–62.

29. Mielke RK, Clemens U, Jens JH, et al. Navigation in knee endoprosthesis implantation: preliminary experience and prospective comparative study with conventional implantation technique. Z Orthop Ihre Grenzgeb 2001;139:109–16.

30. Jenny JY, Boeri C. Navigated implantation of total knee endoprosthesis: a comparative study with conventional instruments. Z Orthop Ihre Grenzgeb 2001;139:117–9.

31. Bonutti PM, Mont MA, McMahon M, et al. Minimally invasive total knee arthroplasty. J Bone Joint Surg Am 2004;86:26–32.

32. Repicci JA. Mini-invasive knee unicompartmental arthroplasty: bone-sparing technique. Surg Technol Int 2003;11:282–6.

33. Dalury DF, Dennis DA. Mini-incision total knee arthroplasty can increase risk of component malalignment. Clin Orthop Relat Res 2005;440:77–81.

34. Insall JN. Choices and compromises in total knee arthroplasty. Clin Orthop Relat Res 1988;226:43–8.

35. Tria AJ, Coon TM. Minimal incision total knee arthroplasty. Clin Orthop Relat Res 2003;416:185–90.

36. Laskin RS. New techniques and concepts in total knee replacement. Clin Orthop Relat Res 2003;416: 151–3.

37. Bonutti PM, Neal DJ, Kestler MA. Minimal incision total knee arthroplasty using the suspended leg technique. Orthopedics 2003;26:899–903.

38. Daubresse F, Vajeu C, Loquet J. Total knee arthroplasty with conventional or navigated technique: comparison of the learning curves in a community hospital. Acta Orthop Belg 2005;71:710–3.

39. King J, Stamper DL, Schaad DC, et al. Minimally invasive total knee arthroplasty compared with traditional total knee arthroplasty: assessment of the learning curve and the post-operative recuperative period. J Bone Joint Surg Am 2007;89:1497–503.

40. Laskin RS. Minimally invasive total knee arthroplasty: the results justify its use. Clin Orthop Relat Res 2005; 440:54–9.

41. Boerger TO, Aglietti P, Mondanelli N, et al. Mini-subvastus versus parapatellar approach in total knee arthroplasty. Clin Orthop Relat Res 2005;440:82–7.

42. Karpman RR, Smith HL. Comparison of the early results of minimally invasive vs standard approaches to total knee arthroplasty: a prospective, randomized study. J Arthroplasty 2008;24(5):681–8.

43. Choong PF, Dowsey MM, Stoney JD. Does accurate anatomical alignment result in better function and quality of life? A prospective randomized

controlled trial comparing conventional and computer-assisted total knee arthroplasty. J Arthroplasty 2008;24(4):560–9.

44. Longstaff LM, Sloan K, Stamp N, et al. Good alignment after total knee arthroplasty leads to faster rehabilitation and better function. J Arthroplasty 2008;24(4):570–8.

45. Scuderi GR, Tenholder M, Capeci C. Surgical approaches in mini-incision total knee arthroplasty. Clin Orthop Relat Res 2004;428:61–7.

46. Hofmann AA, Plaster RL, Murdock LE. Subvastus (southern) approach for primary total knee arthroplasty. Clin Orthop Relat Res 1991;269:70–7.

47. Engh GA, Holt BT, Parks NL. A midvastus muscle-splitting approach for the total knee arthroplasty. J Arthroplasty 1997;12:322–31.

48. Seyler TM, Bonutti PM, Slif DU, et al. Minimally invasive lateral approach to total knee arthroplasty. J Arthroplasty 2007;22(7 Suppl 3):21–6.

49. Labat G. Regional anesthesia: Its technique and clinical applications: regional anesthesia. 2nd edition. Philadelphia: W.B. Saunders; 1924. p. 45–55.

50. Winnie AP, Ramamurthy S, Durrani Z. The inguinal paravascular technique of lumbar plexus anesthesia: the '3-in-1 block'. Anesth Analg 1973;52:989–96.

51. Beck GP. Anterior approach to sciatic nerve block. Anesthesiology 1963;24:222–4.

52. Pham Dang C. Midfemoral block: a new lateral approach to the sciatic nerve. Anesth Analg 1999;88:1426.

53. Meier G. Der kontinuierliche anteriore Ischidicuskatheter (KAI). In: Mehrkens HH, Büttner J (Hrsg). Kontinuerliche periphere Leitungsblockade. Acris Verlag, München, 1999:47–8 [in German].

54. Meier G. Der distale Ischiadicuskatheter (DIK). In: Mehrkens HH, Büttner J (Hrsg). Kontinuerliche periphere Leitungsblockade. Acris Verlag, München, 1999:43–6 [in German].

55. Dalury DF. Observations of the proximal tibia in total knee arthroplasty. Clin Orthop Relat Res 2001;389:150–5.

56. Eckhoff DG, Metzger RG, Vandewalle MV. Malrotation associated with implant alignment technique in total knee arthroplasty. Clin Orthop Relat Res 1995;3211:28–31.

57. Biasca N, Wirth S, Bungartz M. Mechanical accuracy of navigated minimally invasive total knee arthroplasty (MISTKA). Knee 2009;16(1):22–9.

58. Ranawat CS, Insall J, Shine J. Duo-condylar knee arthroplasty: hospital for special surgery design. Clin Orthop Relat Res 1976;120:76–82.

59. Insall JN, Dorr LD, Scott RD, et al. Rationale of the knee society clinical rating system. Clin Orthop Relat Res 1989;248:13–4.

60. Chin PL, Yang KY, Yeo SJ, et al. Randomized control trial comparing radiographic total knee arthroplasty implant placement using computer navigation versus conventional technique. J Arthroplasty 2005;20:618–26.

61. Ewald FC. The knee society total knee arthroplasty roentgenographic evaluation and scoring system. Clin Orthop Relat Res 1989;248:9–12.

62. Yoo JH, Chang CB, Shin KS, et al. Anatomical references to assess the posterior tibial slope in total knee arthroplasty: a comparison of 5 anatomical axes. J Arthroplasty 2008;23(4):586–92.

63. Berger RA, Rubash HE, Seel MJ, et al. Determining the rotational alignment of the femoral component in total knee arthroplasty using the epicondylar axis. Clin Orthop Relat Res 1993;286:40–7.

64. Bauwens K, Matthes G, Wich M, et al. Navigated total knee replacement: a meta-analysis. J Bone Joint Surg Am 2007;89:261–9.

65. Mason JB, Fehring TK, Estok R, et al. Meta-analysis of alignment outcomes in computer-assisted total knee arthroplasty surgery. J Arthroplasty 2007;22(8):1097–106.

66. Jenny JY, Clemens U, Kohler S, et al. Consistency of implantation of a total knee arthroplasty with a non-image-based navigation system. J Arthroplasty 2005;20(7):832–9.

67. Haaker RG, Stockheim M, Kamp M, et al. Computer-assisted navigation increased precision of component placement in total knee arthroplasty. Clin Orthop Relat Res 2005;433:152–9.

68. Molfetta L, Caldo D. Computer navigation versus conventional implantation for varus knee total arthroplasty: a case-control study at 5 years follow-up. Knee 2008;15:75–9.

69. Decking R, Markmann Y, Fuchs J, et al. Leg axis after computer-navigated total knee arthroplasty: a randomized trial comparing computer-navigated and manual implantation. J Arthroplasty 2005;20(3):282–8.

70. Kim YH, Kim JS, Yoon SH. Alignment and orientation of the components in total knee replacement with and without navigation support. J Bone Joint Surg Br 2007;89(4):471–6.

71. Malik MH, Wadia F, Porter ML. Preliminary radiological evaluation of the Vector Vision CT-free knee module for implantation of the LCS knee prosthesis. Knee 2007;14(1):19–21.

72. Siston RA, Patel JJ, Goodman SB, et al. The variability of femoral rotational alignment in total knee arthroplasty. J Bone Joint Surg Am 2005;87:2276–80.

73. Catani F, Biasca N, Ensini A, et al. Alignment deviation between bone resection and final implant positioning in computer-navigated total knee arthroplasty. J Bone Joint Surg Am 2008;90:765–71.

74. Hart R, Janecek M, Chaker A, et al. Total knee arthroplasty implanted with and without kinematic navigation. Int Orthop 2003;27:366–9.

75. Oberst M, Bertsch C, Wurstlin S, et al. CT analysis of leg alignment after conventional versus navigated knee prosthesis implantation. Unfallchirurg 2003; 106:941–8.

76. Olcott CW, Scott RD. The Ranawat Award. Femoral component rotation during total knee arthroplasty. Clin Orthop Relat Res 1999;367:39–42.

77. Chauhan SK, Clark GW, Lloyd S, et al. Computer-assisted total knee replacement: a controlled cadaver study using a multi-parameter quantitative ct assessment of alignment (the Perth CT Protocol). J Bone Joint Surg Br 2004;86:818–23.

78. Siston RA, Giori NJ, Goodman SB, et al. Surgical navigation for total knee arthroplasty: a perspective. J Biomech 2007;40:728–35.

79. Catani F, Biasca N, Ensini A, et al. Tibial and femoral joint line restoration after navigated total knee arthroplasty. J Bone Joint Surg Am 2009 [in review].

80. Van Damme G, Defoort K, Ducoulombier Y, et al. What should the surgeon aim for when performing computer-assisted total knee arthroplasty? J Bone Joint Surg Am 2005;87(Suppl 2):52–8.

81. Tokuhara Y, Kadoya Y, Nakagawa S, et al. The flexion gap in normal knees: an MRI study. J Bone Joint Surg Br 2004;86:1133–6.

82. Todo S, Kadoya Y, Moilanen T, et al. Anteroposterior and rotational movement of the femur during knee flexion. Clin Orthop 1999;362:162–70.

83. Hill PF, Vedi V, Williams A, et al. Tibiofemoral movement 2: the loaded and unloaded living knee studied by MRI. J Bone Joint Surg Br 2000;82: 1196–8.

84. Iwaki H, Pinskerova V, Freeman MAR. Tibiofemoral movement 1: the shapes and relative movement of the femur and tibia in the unloaded cadaver knee. J Bone Joint Surg Br 2000;82:1189–95.

85. Nakagawa S, Kadoya Y, Todo S, et al. Tibiofemoral movement 3: full flexion in the living knee studied by MRI. J Bone Joint Surg Br 2000;82: 1199–200.

86. Moore TH, Meyer MH. Apparatus to position knees for varus-valgus stress roentgenograms. J Bone Joint Surg Am 1977;59:984.

87. Takahashi T, Wada Y, Yamamoto H. Soft tissue balancing with pressure distribution during total knee arthroplasty. J Bone Joint Surg Br 1997;79: 235–9.

88. Stahelin T, Kessler O, Pfirmann C, et al. Fluoroscopy assisted stress radiography for varus-valgus stability assessment in flexion after total knee arthroplasty. J Arthroplasty 2003;18:513–5.

89. Oliver JH, Coughlin LP. Objective knee evaluation using the Genucum knee analysis system: clinical implications. Am J Sports Med 1987;15: 571–8.

90. Wirth S, Biasca N. Joint laxity in navigated total knee arthroplasty. Presented at the 2006 Computer Assisted Orthopaedic Surgery, 5th International Annual Meeting of CAOS, Helsinki, Finland, June 19–22, 2005.

91. Stulberg SD, Yafffe MA, Koo SS. Computer-assisted surgery versus manual total knee arthroplasty: a case-controlled study. J Bone Joint Surg Am 2006;88(4 Supp):47–54.

92. Haas SB, Cook S, Beksac B. Minimally invasive total knee replacement through a mini midvastus approach: a comparative study. Clin Orthop Relat Res 2004;428:68–73.

93. Haas SB, Manitta MA, Burdick P. Minimally invasive total knee arthroplasty: the mini midvastus approach. Clin Orthop Relat Res 2006;452: 112–6.

94. Lingard EA, Katz JN, Wright RJ, et al. Validity and responsiveness of the knee society clinical rating system in comparison with the SF-36 and WOMAC. J Bone Joint Surg Am 2001;83(12): 1856–64.

Index

Note: Page numbers of article titles are in **boldface** type.

Orthop Clin N Am 40 (2009) 565–568
doi:10.1016/S0030-5898(09)00081-9
0030-5898/09/$ – see front matter © 2009 Elsevier Inc. All rights reserved.

orthopedic.theclinics.com

United States Postal Service

Statement of Ownership, Management, and Circulation
(All Periodicals Publications Except Requestor Publications)

1. Publication Title	2. Publication Number	3. Filing Date
Orthopedic Clinics of North America	9 5 0 - 9 2 0	9/15/09

4. Issue Frequency	5. Number of Issues Published Annually	6. Annual Subscription Price
Jan, Apr, Jul, Oct	4	$244.00

7. Complete Mailing Address of Known Office of Publication (Not printer) (Street, city, county, state, and ZIP+4®)

Elsevier Inc.
360 Park Avenue South
New York, NY 10010-1710

Contact Person
Stephen Bushing
Telephone (Include area code)
215-239-3688

8. Complete Mailing Address of Headquarters or General Business Office of Publisher (Not printer)

Elsevier Inc. 360 Park Avenue South, New York, NY 10010-1710

9. Full Names and Complete Mailing Addresses of Publisher, Editor, and Managing Editor (Do not leave blank)

Publisher (Name and complete mailing address)

John Schrefer, Elsevier, Inc., 1600 John F. Kennedy Blvd. Suite 1800, Philadelphia, PA 19103-2899

Editor (Name and complete mailing address)

Deb Dellapena, Elsevier, Inc., 1600 John F. Kennedy Blvd. Suite 1800, Philadelphia, PA 19103-2899

Managing Editor (Name and complete mailing address)

Catherine Bewick, Elsevier, Inc., 1600 John F. Kennedy Blvd. Suite 1800, Philadelphia, PA 19103-2899

10. Owner (Do not leave blank. If the publication is owned by a corporation, give the name and address of the corporation immediately followed by the names and addresses of all stockholders owning or holding 1 percent or more of the total amount of stock. If not owned by a corporation, give the names and addresses of the individual owners. If owned by a partnership or other unincorporated firm, give its name and address as well as those of each individual owner. If the publication is published by a nonprofit organization, give its name and address.)

Full Name	Complete Mailing Address
Wholly owned subsidiary of	4520 East-West Highway
Reed/Elsevier, US holdings	Bethesda, MD 20814

11. Known Bondholders, Mortgagees, and Other Security Holders Owning or Holding 1 Percent or More of Total Amount of Bonds, Mortgages, or Other Securities. If none, check box ☐ None

Full Name	Complete Mailing Address
N/A	

12. Tax Status (For completion by nonprofit organizations authorized to mail at nonprofit rates) (Check one)
The purpose, function, and nonprofit status of this organization and the exempt status for federal income tax purposes:
☐ Has Not Changed During Preceding 12 Months
☐ Has Changed During Preceding 12 Months (Publisher must submit explanation of change with this statement)

PS Form 3526, September 2007 (Page 1 of 3 (Instructions Page 3)) PSN 7530-01-000-9931 PRIVACY NOTICE: See our Privacy policy in www.usps.com

---

13. Publication Title		14. Issue Date for Circulation Data Below
Orthopedic Clinics of North America		April 2009

15. Extent and Nature of Circulation		Average No. Copies Each Issue During Preceding 12 Months	No. Copies of Single Issue Published Nearest to Filing Date
a. Total Number of Copies (Net press run)		2734	2337
b. Paid Circulation (By Mail and Outside the Mail)	(1) Mailed Outside-County Paid Subscriptions Stated on PS Form 3541. (Include paid distribution above nominal rate, advertiser's proof copies, and exchange copies)	1030	892
	(2) Mailed In-County Paid Subscriptions Stated on PS Form 3541 (Include paid distribution above nominal rate, advertiser's proof copies, and exchange copies)		
	(3) Paid Distribution Outside the Mails Including Sales Through Dealers and Carriers, Street Vendors, Counter Sales, and Other Paid Distribution Outside USPS®	871	736
	(4) Paid Distribution by Other Classes Mailed Through the USPS (e.g. First-Class Mail®)		
c. Total Paid Distribution (Sum of 15b (1), (2), (3), and (4))		1901	1628
d. Free or Nominal Rate Distribution (By Mail and Outside the Mail)	(1) Free or Nominal Rate Outside-County Copies Included on PS Form 3541	104	102
	(2) Free or Nominal Rate In-County Copies Included on PS Form 3541		
	(3) Free or Nominal Rate Copies Mailed at Other Classes Through the USPS (e.g. First-Class Mail)		
	(4) Free or Nominal Rate Distribution Outside the Mail (Carriers or other means)		
e. Total Free or Nominal Rate Distribution (Sum of 15d (1), (2), (3) and (4))		104	102
f. Total Distribution (Sum of 15c and 15e)		2005	1730
g. Copies not Distributed (See instructions to publishers #4 (page #3))		729	607
h. Total (Sum of 15f and g)		2734	2337
i. Percent Paid (15c divided by 15f times 100)		94.81%	94.10%

16. Publication of Statement of Ownership
If the publication is a general publication, publication of this statement is required. Will be printed in the October 2009 issue of this publication. ☐ Publication not required

17. Signature and Title of Editor, Publisher, Business Manager, or Owner

Jean Fereluci — Executive Director of Subscription Services

Date
September 15, 2009

I certify that all information furnished on this form is true and complete. I understand that anyone who furnishes false or misleading information on this form or who omits material or information requested on the form may be subject to criminal sanctions (including fines and imprisonment) and/or civil sanctions (including civil penalties).

PS Form 3526, September 2007 (Page 2 of 3)

Printed and bound by CPI Group (UK) Ltd, Croydon, CR0 4YY

03/10/2024

01040362-0009